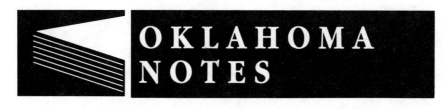

Clinical Sciences Review for Medical Licensure
Developed at
The University of Oklahoma College of Medicine

Ronald S. Krug, *Series Editor*

Suitable Review for:
United States Medical Licensing Examination
(USMLE), Step 2

Springer
New York
Berlin
Heidelberg
Barcelona
Budapest
Hong Kong
London
Milan
Paris
Santa Clara
Singapore
Tokyo

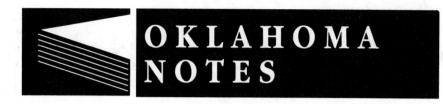

OKLAHOMA NOTES

Family Medicine

Second Edition

Jeffrey G. Hirsch

Rita R. Claudet
Technical Editor

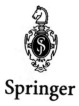

Springer

Jeffrey G. Hirsch, M.D.
Metro Medical Associates
Family Practice Medicine
120 North Robinson
First National Center Arcade
Oklahoma City, OK 73102 USA

Library of Congress Cataloging-in-Publication Data
Hirsch, Jeffrey G.
    Family medicine / Jeffrey G. Hirsch ; Rita R. Claudet, technical
editor. — 2nd ed.
        p.   cm. — (Oklahoma notes)
    Includes bibliographical references.
    ISBN 0-387-94638-1 (pbk. : alk. paper)
    1. Family medicine—Outlines, syllabi, etc. I. Title.
II. Series.
RC59.H55   1996
616—dc20   96-1058

Printed on acid-free paper.

Production managed by Robert Wexler; manufacturing supervised by Joe Quatela.
Camera-ready copy prepared by the author.
Printed and bound by Edwards Brothers, Inc., Ann Arbor, MI.
Printed in the United States of America.

9 8 7 6 5 4 3 2 1

ISBN 0-387-94638-1 Springer-Verlag New York Berlin Heidelberg   SPIN 10522850

Preface to the Oklahoma Notes

The intent of the Oklahoma Notes is to provide students with a set of texts that present the basic information of the general medical school curriculum in such a manner that the content is clear, concise and can be readily absorbed.

The basic outline format that has made the Oklahoma Notes extremely popular when preparing for standardized examinations has been retained in all the texts. The educational goals for these materials are first to help organize thinking about given categories of information, and second, to present the information in a format that assists in learning. The information that students retain best is that which has been repeated often, and has been actively recalled. The outline format has always been used in the Oklahoma Notes because students have reported to us that it allows them to cover subsequent parts of the outline, and use the topic heading as a trigger to recall the information under the heading. They then can uncover the material and ascertain whether they have recalled the information correctly.

This second edition of the Clinical Series of the Oklahoma Notes represents a major refinement of the first edition. A number of issues have been addressed to make the texts more efficient, effective and "user friendly." These include:

- Correction of technical errors.
- Addition of new material that has been reported since the first editions were published.
- Standard presentation of materials in all texts to make information more accessible to the student.
- Review questions written in standardized format. These questions reflect the major issues of the sections of the texts.

We hope these are helpful to you in your educational progress and preparation for required examinations.

Ronald S. Krug, Ph.D.
Series Editor

Preface

Studying for licensure examinations is like eating a twelve course meal: if you try and do it in five minutes, it will make you sick. As you prepare, pace yourself, don't memorize but review, and, most importantly, a few days before the examination, try and get some rest.

I don't think I've ever heard of a soul who looked forward to this examination, and I can assure you no one has ever walked out saying "What a wonderful experience." Think of this ordeal as a rite of passage and try to remember that most of you will make it through.

I'd like to thank Dr. Ron Krug for his continued support and guidance, not only in the preparation of this text, but through the years.

Additional thanks to Dr. Rita Claudet for continued suggestions and editing of this text.

Good luck in your studies and remember what Winston Churchill said, "Never, never, never, give up!"

Jeffrey G. Hirsch, M.D.
Oklahoma City

Contents

DAY 1.

DAY 2.

DAY 3.

DAY 4.

DAY 5.

To Marilyn and Emanuel,
who encouraged me to dream.
To Regina, Hannah and Adam,
who dream with me.

I. PAPULOSQUAMOUS ERUPTIONS

    A. *Psoriasis*

        1. DEFINITION

            a. An acute or chronic, unpredictable disease characterized by erythematous plaques with superimposed silvery scales of unknown etiology.

            b. Genetic predisposition, perhaps an autosomal dominant inheritance.

        2. DIAGNOSIS

            a. Check for triggering situations

                (1) Stress

                (2) Nonspecific physical trauma

                (3) Drugs

                    (a) Lithium

                    (b) Beta blockers

                    (c) Following discontinuation of systemic glucocorticoids

                (4) Infections

                    Streptococcal

            b. By visual inspection of commonly affected area such as scalp, elbows, knees and buttock but lesions can occur anywhere.

            c. Ridges and pits in nails.

            d. Auspitz's sign

                A punctate bleeding site when the scale is removed.

            e. Biopsy may be necessary.

            f. 5-10% of patients have joint pain.

            g. **Generalized pustular psoriasis**

                A potentially life-threatening disorder that *may* occur following the discontinuation of systemic glucocorticoids.

        3. TREATMENT

            a. Mild to moderate disease

                (1) Skin lubricants, moderate sun exposure and topical steroids.

                (2) Keratolytic agents

                (3) **Don't use fluorinated steroids on the face**.

                (4) Coal tar shampoo and steroid lotions for the scalp.

                (5) Intralesional injection with steroids of highly visible lesions.

            b. Severe disease

                (1) Ultraviolet B (UV-B) alone or with either coal tar or anthralin

                (2) Ultraviolet A (UV-A) combined with oral or topical psoralens

                (3) Superficial X-ray

                (4) Methotrexate

    B. Fungal infections

        1. Dermatophytes

            a. DEFINITION

                (1) Fungi that infect the skin, the hair and the nails

(2) Skin lesions are characterized by an erythematous rash with a distinct vesicular, papular, or scaly border and central clearing.

    (a) *Tinea capitis*
- Scalp lesions with central hair loss
- Contagious
- Etiology
  - *Microsporum canis*
  - *Trichophyton tonsurans*

    (b) *Tinea cruris*
- "Jock itch" with lesions affecting the inguinal folds
- Etiology
  - *Trichophyton rubrum*
  - *Epidermophyton floccosum*

    (c) *Tinea pedis*
- "Athlete's foot"
- Etiology
  - *Trichophyton mentagrophytes*
  - *Trichophyton rubrum*

    (d) *Tinea corporis*
- "Ringworm"
- Lesions affecting face, trunk and extremities
- Etiology
  - *Trichophyton rubrum*

    (e) *Tinea unguium*
- Onychomycosis
- A fungal infection of the nail plate, nail bed or both

b. DIAGNOSIS
- (1) KOH prep of lesions + for septa and branched hyphae.
- (2) Only *Microsporum* species fluoresce with Wood's light.

c. TREATMENT
- (1) For *Tinea cruris, pedis,* and *corporis* topical clotrimazole or miconazole
- (2) For widespread or resistant lesions, and for the treatment of *Tinea unguium* and *Tinea capitis* in adults, systemic fluconazole or ketoconazole.

2. *Tinea versicolor*

a. DEFINITION
- (1) A common superficial mycosis with discrete and confluent patches or plaques involving sebum rich areas of the back, shoulders and chest.
- (2) Etiology
  - *Malassezia furfur*

  b. DIAGNOSIS
    (1) The lesions are white on sun-exposed areas and brown or red-brown on covered areas. Easy to diagnose in the summer.
    (2) KOH prep
      + budding yeast forms and club-shaped hyphae
  c. TREATMENT
    (1) Scrub lesions with 2.5% selenium sulfide shampoo for two to three weeks.
    (2) Topical antifungals, clotrimazole or miconazole for two weeks
 3. *Candidiasis*
  a. DEFINITION
    (1) Erythematous lesions on mucous membranes or moist areas of the skin.
    (2) Predisposing conditions that encourage Candida growth
      (a) Diabetes mellitus
      (b) Obesity
      (c) Long-term use of oral contraceptives
      (d) Following the use of broad-spectrum antibiotics
      (e) Immunosuppression
    (3) Etiology
      Candida albicans causes the majority of infections.
    (4) Oral Candidiasis is also called Thrush.
    (5) Candida vaginitis is the most common form of yeast infection.
  b. DIAGNOSIS
    (1) KOH prep
      + for budding yeast-like cells.
    (2) Gram stain
      + for yeast forms.
  c. TREATMENT
    (1) Oral lesions, nystatin oral suspension, or clotrimazole troche, or systemic antifungal fluconazole.
    (2) Vaginal lesions, miconazole, or clotrimazole or terconazole cream or suppositories. For resistant or recurrent cases, systemic fluconazole.

II. PYODERMAS
 A. *Folliculitis*
  1. DEFINITION
    a. Small erythematous papules or pustules involving the hair follicles *without* involvement of surrounding skin or dermis.
    b. Etiology
      Usually *Staphylococcus aureus*

2. DIAGNOSIS
   a. Close examination of the lesions reveal a hair at the center of the papule or pustule.
   b. Laboratory
      (1) Gram stain
      (2) Culture of lesion
3. TREATMENT
   a. Hot compresses for small localized lesions
   b. Antibiotic therapy for multiple or recurrent infection
      (1) Antibiotic therapy is initiated with a beta-lactamase resistant antibiotic
      (2) **Staphylococcal infections are resistant to penicillin.**

B. *Furuncle*
   1. DEFINITION
      a. "A boil" An *invasive* or more extensive infection involving the follicle or sebaceous gland which extends into the subcutaneous tissues.
      b. **Hidradenitis suppurativa**
         Staphylococcal infection involving the *apocrine glands* of the groin and axilla
   2. DIAGNOSIS
      a. Localized swelling
      b. Erythema
      c. Pain
      d. ± itching
      e. Pain to palpation
      f. Laboratory
         (1) Gram stain
         (2) Culture of lesion
   3. TREATMENT
      a. Hot compresses for smaller localized lesions
      b. Incise and drain larger lesions
      c. Antibiotic therapy is initiated with a beta-lactamase resistant antibiotic

C. *Carbuncle*
   1. DEFINITION
      a. A painful, deeper, indurated lesion larger than a furuncle that is loculated, usually with multiple drainage sites.
      b. Think multiple, *interconnected* furuncles
      c. Etiology
         Staphylococcus aureus
   2. DIAGNOSIS
      a. Fever
      b. Pain
      c. Leukocytosis
      d. ± bacteremia

e. Laboratory
  (1) Gram stain
  (2) Culture of lesion
3. TREATMENT
  a. Incise and drain
  b. Antibiotic therapy is initiated with a beta-lactamase resistant antibiotic

D. *Impetigo*
  1. DEFINITION
    A superficial, intradermal, vesiculopustular infection that is highly contagious.
  2. DIAGNOSIS
    a. **Nonbullous Impetigo**
      (1) Etiology
        (a) Most commonly Group A beta-hemolytic *Streptococci.*
        (b) *Staphylococcus aureus* infection is much less common.
        (c) Mixed cultures may occur.
      (2) Most common in children
      (3) Frequently seen on the face or at trauma site
      (4) The early lesions are an erythematous macule or papule. Weeping lesions form painless, shallow ulcers with *"honey-colored crusts"*
      (5) Acute glomerulonephritis may occur when nephritogenic strains of Group A streptococci are the etiology of infection.
    b. **Bullous Impetigo**
      Usually a *Staphylococcus aureus,* impetigo that progresses rapidly from a small erythematous papule to a large flaccid-thin roofed bulla.
    c. **Ecthyma**
      A deeper, ulcerated, lower extremity impetigo associated with lymphangitis.
    d. Laboratory
      (1) Gram stain and wound cultures
        + for *Streptococci* and/or *Staphylococci*
  3. TREATMENT
    a. Debride the lesions of the crusts
    b. For single or small, localized lesions, mupirocin
    c. For widespread lesions, systemic antibiotic therapy
      (1) Beta-lactamase resistant antibiotic
      (2) **Avoid erythromycin because of widespread resistance.**

E. *Cellulitis*
  1. DEFINITION
    a. A rapidly spreading infection of the skin, dermis and subcutaneous tissues.
    b. Etiology
      Staphylococcal and streptococcal organisms predominate

    c. Different clinical entities and/or etiology of infection are identified by location
        (1) Facial cellulitis and cellulitis of the upper extremity especially in children consider *Hemophilus influenzae.*
        (2) Cellulitis of the lower extremity consider Group A, beta-hemolytic *Streptococci. Staphylococcus aureus* much less common.
        (3) **Erysipelas**
            (a) "St. Anthony's Fire", *a superficial cellulitis* with marked involvement of the lymphatics.
            (b) Etiology
                Group A, beta-hemolytic *Streptococci.*
        (4) **Periorbital cellulitis**
            (a) Proptosis and painful ophthalmoplegia secondary to extension of infection from contiguous structures that surround the orbit.
            (b) Immediate treatment may prevent serious complications such as brain abscess, meningitis or cavernous sinus thrombosis
        (5) Cellulitis secondary to animal bites consider *Pasteurella multocida.*
        (6) Cellulitis secondary to ulcerations consider gram-negative rods and anaerobes.

2. DIAGNOSIS
    a. Erythematous lesion that is swollen and tender with an *indefinite border* that may involve a large area of the skin.
    b. Pain, swelling and fever, ± chills
    c. A rapidly spreading infection, ± lymphangitis and regional lymphadenopathy
    d. Laboratory
        (1) Elevated white count
        (2) ± + cultures about half the time.
    e. **Erysipelas**
        (1) Seen most often in children and elderly
        (2) An erythematous, warm, indurated, plaque with *sharp borders.*
        (3) The face is most commonly involved.
        (4) Fever is common
        (5) + lymphatic involvement
            Edema and "*peau d'orange*" appearance.
        (6) Lesions don't itch, they hurt.
        (7) Laboratory
            ± cultures + for *Streptococci*

3. TREATMENT
    a. Dependent upon organism and severity of disease.
        (1) Mild infections
            (a) Penicillin for Streptococci
            (b) Cephalosporins for *Staphylococci*

(2) Amoxicillin-clavulanic acid for bites.

(3) Severe infections require hospitalization with IV meds dependent upon organism isolated and its antibiotic sensitivity.

III. VIRAL INFECTION

A. *Herpes simplex*

1. DEFINITION

a. A *viral infection* characterized by grouped vesicles on an erythematous base. These lesions rupture to form painful ulcerations.

b. **HSV 1 and HSV 2 can be associated with severe, life-threatening infections in immunocompromised patients.**

c. Etiology

(1) *Herpesvirus hominis*

(a) *TYPE 1 (HSV 1)*

▸ The common *fever blister* or *cold sore*.

• Predisposing factors

○ Stress

○ Febrile infection

○ Exposure to UV radiation (usually sunlight)

▸ Usual 10-14 day course.

(b) *TYPE 2 (HSV 2)*

▸ A sexually transmitted disease.

▸ Recurrent genital herpes is almost always HSV2.

▸ **"Asymptomatic shedding"**.

▸ The usual 10-14 day course may extend several weeks.

2. DIAGNOSIS

a. Visual identification confirmed with Tzanck smear.

+ smear reveals multinucleated giant cells.

b. Viral cultures + 80-90% in early lesions.

c. Antigen detection using monoclonal antibodies.

3. TREATMENT

Acyclovir

IV. INFESTATIONS

A. *Scabies*

1. DEFINITION

a. A pruritic, contagious infestation caused by *Sarcoptes scabiei*.

b. Also known as "seven year itch"

2. DIAGNOSIS

a. Generalized itching that is worse at night

b. Scrape lesions and examine under oil mount slides or KOH preps

3. TREATMENT
   a. Always treat patient *and* close contacts
   b. Permethrin cream or lindane, lotion, cream or shampoo
   c. Wash clothing and bedding

B. *Pediculosis*
   1. DEFINITION
      a. "Human lice" or "crabs"
      b. Intensely pruritic and a very contagious infestation.
      c. Etiologies
         (1) *Phthirus pubis*
             Pubic or crab louse
         (2) *Pediculus humanus corporis*
             Body louse
         (3) *Pediculus capitis*
             Head louse
      d. Nits = eggs
         (1) The nits of head and pubic lice attach to the hair shafts.
         (2) Body lice eggs are laid in the clothing.
   2. DIAGNOSIS
      Visual identification with hand lens of lice or nits.
   3. TREATMENT
      a. Always treat patient *and* close contacts.
      b. Permethrin cream or lindane, lotion, cream or shampoo.
      c. Wash clothing and bedding.

V. DERMATITIS
   A. *Contact Dermatitis*
   1. DEFINITION
      a. A skin eruption characterized by erythema, papules, vesicles, vesiculobullous lesions, excoriation and sometimes edema.
      b. Etiologies
         (1) *Irritant variety*
             Noxious substances such as acids, alkali, or solvents produce inflammation *without* provoking a specific antibody response.
         (2) *Allergic contact dermatitis*
             (a) Specific T-cell antibodies are generated against the allergen.
             (b) Examples: poison ivy, oak and sumac
   2. DIAGNOSIS
      A good history and visual identification of lesions.
   3. TREATMENT
      a. Antihistamines

  b. Potent topical steroids
  c. Systemic steroids
B. *Seborrheic Dermatitis*
  1. DEFINITION
    a. A common superficial inflammatory disorder of the skin involving the hairy areas of the body, most commonly the face and head.
    b. Etiology
      Unknown, but *Pityrosporum ovale*, a lipophilic yeast, may contribute.
  2. DIAGNOSIS
    a. Erythema and scaling in patches or plaques over the hairy areas of the body. The margins are indistinct.
    b. Pruritus is common.
      (1) **Cradle cap**
        Seborrheic dermatitis of scalp in infants.
      (2) **Seborrhea sicca**
        Dandruff, the most common form of seborrhea.
  3. TREATMENT
    a. Infants
      (1) It will usually disappear within the first year.
      (2) Sulfur shampoos and apply 1% hydrocortisone lotion.
    b. Adults
      (1) Mid-potency steroid lotions
      (2) Sulfur containing, or selenium sulfide 2%, or chloroxine 2% shampoos.
C. *Stasis Dermatitis*
  1. DEFINITION
    a. Chronic noninflammatory edema of the lower legs secondary to venous valve failure.
      (1) Initial edema→itching→ excoriation followed by weeping, crusting lesions
      (2) Stasis ulcers may also form
  2. DIAGNOSIS
    a. Usually distal third of the leg
    b. Reddish-brown postinflammatory hyperpigmentation with associated edema.
  3. TREATMENT
    a. Elevation
    b. Jobst stockings
    c. Exercise
    d. Topical steroids or skin lubricants depending upon dermatitis present.
    e. Treat stasis ulcer with appropriate antibiotics.

VI. VASCULAR DISORDERS

A. *Acute Urticaria*
1. DEFINITION
   a. "Hives" These lesions form the classic *wheal* or *wheal and flare*.
   b. Etiologies
      (1) An IgE-mediated histamine release from mast cells
      (2) Idiosyncratic drug reaction.
2. DIAGNOSIS
   Pruritic lesions, light pink macules surrounded by an erythematous halo that may be larger than the wheal.
3. TREATMENT
   a. Antihistamines
   b. Systemic steroids for resistant cases.

B. *Erythema Multiforme*
1. DEFINITION
   a. An acute, self-limiting inflammatory disorder of the skin and mucous membranes.
   b. Etiologies
      (1) **50% idiopathic**
      (2) Hypersensitivity Response
         (a) *Herpes simplex*
         (b) *Mycoplasma pneumoniae*
         (c) Antibiotics
         (d) Anticonvulsants
         (e) Aspirin
   c. **Erythema multiforme minor**
      Rash ± one mucous membrane site
   d. **Erythema multiforme major**
      (1) *Stevens-Johnson Syndrome*
         (a) Severe involvement of skin and mucous membranes
         (b) Multiple organ systems ± involvement
2. DIAGNOSIS
   a. **Target lesions**
      A classic rash characterized by central erythema, often with a central vesicle surrounded by normal appearing skin and an outer ring of erythema.
   b. Lesions on the face, palms, soles, and extensor surfaces of arms and legs.
3. TREATMENT
   a. Attention and treatment to underlying disease
   b. Withdrawal of offending agent.
   c. Systemic steroids may be helpful, if not contraindicated.
   d. Stevens-Johnson Syndrome
      Hospitalization

C. *Erythema Nodosum*
1. DEFINITION
    a. A rash characterized by *bilateral, painful*, erythematous nodules typically over the anterior tibia.
    b. Etiologies
        (1) **Idiopathic**
        (2) Infections
            (a) Streptococcal infections
            (b) Mononucleosis
            (c) Tuberculosis
        (3) Medications
            (a) Sulfa drugs
            (b) Oral contraceptives
        (4) Other
            (a) Sarcoidosis
            (b) Certain malignancies
            (c) Pregnancy
2. DIAGNOSIS
    Bilateral, painful, nonsuppurative, red nodules typically over the anterior tibia.
3. TREATMENT
    a. Remove the offending agent
    b. Treatment with antibiotics, if appropriate.
    c. NSAIDs are the helpful.

VII. **HYPERPLASIA**
A. *Condylomata Acuminata*
1. DEFINITION
    a. "Venereal warts"
    b. Etiology
        Human papilloma virus
    c. Highly contagious with incubation 1-6 months
    d. **Condyloma lata is the rash associated with secondary syphilis. It has nothing to do with Condyloma acuminata.**
2. DIAGNOSIS
    a. A lesion that may appear soft and somewhat flat or have a sessile cauliflower-like appearance.
    b. Lesions can occur on the penis, scrotum, rectum, labia, vagina, cervix, urethra, mouth and throat.
3. TREATMENT
    a. Podofilox or podophyllum in tincture of Benzoin
    b. Cryotherapy

VIII. NEOPLASIA, BENIGN
A. *Nevi*
1. DEFINITION
a. **Intradermal nevi**
(1) The most common nevi composed of cells related to melanocytes, forming dermal nests and strands.
(2) **They don't give rise to melanoma.**
b. **Junctional nevi**
(1) Nevus cells form nests of cells at the junction of the epidermis and the dermis.
(2) **They rarely give rise to melanoma.**
c. **Compound nevi**
Containing elements of *both* intradermal and junctional nevi.
2. DIAGNOSIS
a. A pigmented lesion of the skin that can occur on any area of the body.
b. It may be a flat or raised lesion.
3. TREATMENT
a. If there is any doubt about it's etiology remove it and check the histopathology.
b. **On any worrisome pigmented lesion, *always, always, always* biopsy it and check the histopathology.**

IX. NEOPLASIA, PREMALIGNANT
A. *Actinic Keratosis*
1. DEFINITION
The most common *premalignant* skin lesion secondary to chronic sun exposure.
2. DIAGNOSIS
a. These slightly raised skin lesions occur on chronically sun-damaged skin.
b. Their surfaces are rough to touch and have a slight silvery scale.
3. TREATMENT
Cryotherapy or electrodesiccation.
B. *Leukoplakia*
1. DEFINITION
A whitish thickening on a mucous membranes secondary to sun, tobacco, or trauma.
2. DIAGNOSIS
Biopsy is the only appropriate diagnostic procedure.
3. TREATMENT
Cryotherapy, laser, electrodesiccation or surgery depending upon the lesion's size.

X. NEOPLASIA, MALIGNANT

A. *Basal Cell Carcinoma*

1. DEFINITION
   a. A malignant tumor arising from the basal cells and/or appendages of the epidermis.
   b. *The most common skin cancer*.

2. DIAGNOSIS
   a. Classically, a pearly, translucent, smooth papule with rolled edges and surface telangiectasia on chronically sun-exposed skin.
   b. Most lesions are diagnosed on the head and neck of older patients.
   c. **Biopsy is the only appropriate diagnostic procedure.**

3. TREATMENT
   Electrodesiccation and curettage, excision, laser therapy, or cryotherapy.

4. PROGNOSIS
   a. Excellent but 50% have a recurrence within five years
   b. Metastatic disease is rare.

B. *Squamous Cell Carcinoma*

1. DEFINITION
   a. A malignant skin lesion arising from the cells above the basal layer.
   b. The second most common skin cancer.
   c. **Bowen's disease**
      Epidermal squamous cell carcinoma *in situ*.

2. DIAGNOSIS
   a. A hyperkeratotic papule or nodule sometimes ulcerated on sun-exposed skin.
   b. An actinic keratosis is a common precursor.
   c. **Biopsy is the only appropriate diagnostic procedure.**

3. TREATMENT
   Electrodesiccation and curettage, excision, laser or cryotherapy.

4. PROGNOSIS
   a. Good
   b. Local recurrence possible with ↑ lesions more likely to metastasize than a basal cell

C. *Melanoma*

1. DEFINITION
   a. Malignant melanoma the most dangerous cutaneous malignancy. It is usually an invasive, pigmented tumor of the skin with a high metastatic potential.
   b. **Melanoma is a deadly tumor.**
   c. Clinical entities
      (1) *Superficial spreading melanoma*............... **≈70% of pts.**
      (2) *Nodular melanoma*..................................≈15% of pts.
      (3) *Acral lentiginous*.................................≈2-8% of pts.
      (4) *Lentigo maligna*..................................≈4-10% of pts.

2. DIAGNOSIS
   a. **The "ABCD" of malignant transformation**
      (1) A = Asymmetry
      (2) B = Border irregularity
      (3) C = Color change
      (4) D = Diameter enlargement
   b. **Surgical biopsy is the only appropriate diagnostic procedure.**
3. TREATMENT
   a. Excision of the lesion with margins.
      (1) Therapeutic lymphadenectomy
         Dissection of regional lymph nodes if clinically positive nodes.
      (2) Prophylactic lymphadenectomy
         Dissection of regional lymph nodes if there are clinically negative nodes
         is controversial.
   b. Chemotherapy has not been proven effective.
      There are many experimental protocols under investigation.
   c. Immunotherapy is under investigation.
4. STAGING
   a. *Clark's levels of thickness*
      (1) Level I........In situ.
      (2) Level II......Invasive into the papillary dermis.
      (3) Level III.....Fills the papillary dermis, but doesn't invade the reticular dermis
      (4) Level IV.....Invasion into the reticular dermis.
      (5) Level V......Invasion into the subcutaneous fat.
   b. *Clinical Staging System* (American Joint Committee on Cancer)
      (1) IA.............Localized melanoma <0.75 mm (Clark level II)
      (2) IB.............Localized melanoma <0.76 to 1.5 mm (Clark level III)
      (3) IIA............Localized melanoma 1.5 to 4 mm (Clark level IV)
      (4) IIB............Localized melanoma >4 mm (Clark level V)
      (5) III.............Limited nodal metastases involving only *one* regional group of
         lymph nodes or less than 5 intransit metastases without
         nodal metastases.
      (6) IV.............Advanced regional metastases or distant metastases.
5. PROGNOSIS
   a. **The deeper the penetration the worse the prognosis.**
   b. Primary lesions < .76 mm......................10-year survival of >90%.
   c. + nodes ↓ survival rate to 13-40%
   d. There are only rare cases of survival with stage IV disease.

I. DISEASES OF THE OUTER EYE
    A. *Strabismus*
        1. DEFINITION
            a. A deviation of the normal position of the eye.
                (1) Esotropia
                    Deviation of the eye inward toward the nose.
                (2) Exotropia
                    Deviation of the eye outward away from the nose.
                (3) Hypertropia
                    Vertical deviation on the eye.
        2. TREATMENT
            a. Referral for corrective lenses
            b. Surgery.
    B. *Amblyopia*
        1. DEFINITION
            A reduction in visual acuity in an otherwise anatomically normal eye.
        2. TREATMENT
            a. "Patching" of the lazy eye
            b. Referral to an ophthalmologist for any corrective surgery.

II. REFRACTIVE ERRORS
    A. DEFINITIONS
        1. *Myopia* ....Nearsightedness
        2. *Hyperopia* ....Farsightedness
        3. *Astigmatism*.......An uneven curvature of the cornea
    B. TREATMENT
        Referral for corrective lenses

III. DISEASES OF THE LIDS
    A. *Hordeolum*
        1. DEFINITION
            a. "A sty"
            b. A localized follicular infection of an eyelash or sebaceous gland in the lid margin.
        2. DIAGNOSIS
            Usually a *Staphylococcus* sp. causing a small boil-like lesion and an erythematous
            eyelid.
        3. TREATMENT
            a. Hot compresses.
            b. Topical antibiotic drops or ointment.
            c. I&D by ophthalmologist if it doesn't resolve in two weeks.

B. *Chalazion*
 1. DEFINITION
  A *localized nodule* on the lid representing a chronic swelling *not* associated with conjunctivitis.
 2. DIAGNOSIS
  Rubbery, cystic lesion of the lid non-tender to palpation.
 3. TREATMENT
  a. Hot compress to decrease size
  b. Topical antibiotics *don't* work
  c. Systemic antibiotics may be indicated
  d. I&D lesion by curettage if the lesion persists

C. *Blepharitis*
 1. DEFINITION
  a. A *chronic* lid inflammation of the glands surrounding the eyelashes.
   (1) **Allergic (Seborrheic) Blepharitis**
    A type of contact dermatitis
   (2) **Staphylococcal Blepharitis**
    The most common infection of the outer eye
 2. DIAGNOSIS
  a. An erythematous lid with or without scaling
  b. There is *no* ulceration.
  c. It is usually bilateral.
 3. TREATMENT
  a. Removal of offending agents
  b. Topical antibiotics
  c. Hot compresses
  d. For severe infection, systemic antibiotics
  e. It frequently exacerbates.

IV. **DISEASES OF THE CONJUNCTIVA**
 A. *Conjunctivitis*
  1. DEFINITION
   a. An infection of the palpebral and/or bulbar conjunctiva.
   b. Most common etiologies
    (1) Bacterial
     (a) *Staphylococcus aureus*
     (b) *Streptococcus pneumoniae*
     (c) *Hemophilus influenzae*
     (d) *Neisseria* sp.

(2) Viral

    (a) Adenoviruses

        Epidemic Keratoconjunctivitis (pink eye) is highly contagious and spread by person-to-person contact or fomites.

    (b) *Herpes simplex*

(3) Chlamydia

    The most common cause of *infectious* neonatal conjunctivitis.

(4) Noninfectious

    (a) Allergic

    (b) Chemical

        The 1% buffered silver nitrate solution placed in the eyes of newborn babies to prevent *Neisseria* infection is the most common cause of neonatal conjunctivitis.

c. **Systemic diseases may manifest signs and symptoms in the eye.**

    (1) Stevens-Johnson syndrome

    (2) Gout

    (3) Carcinoid

    (4) Sarcoidosis

    (5) Thyroid

2. DIAGNOSIS

    a. A good history is mandatory.

    b. A "red eye". There's always erythema.

    c. Dependent on organism

        (1) Tearing

        (2) Matting

        (3) Burning

        (4) Pruritus

        (5) Exudate

        (6) Lid edema

        (7) Photophobia

    d. Laboratory

        (1) Gram stain

        (2) Giemsa stain

        (3) Conjunctival culture

3. TREATMENT

    a. Dependent upon etiology

        (1) Bacterial

            (a) Topical antibiotics.

            (b) *Neisseria* spp.

                IV or IM antibiotics

(2) Viral

    (a) Adenovirus is self-limiting.

    (b) Herpes

        ▸ Topical idoxuridine

        ▸ Topical and/or oral acyclovir

    (c) Chlamydia

        ▸ Doxycycline

        ▸ Erythromycin in children

(3) Allergic

    (a) Antihistamines

    (b) Topical vasoconstrictors.

(4) Chemical

    (a) Removal of noxious substance via irrigation.

    (b) Antihistamines

    (c) Guard against secondary bacterial infection.

  b. **Be careful using topical steroids on the eye, especially if you suspect HSV or other infectious agents.**

V. DISEASES OF THE LENS

  A. *Cataracts*

    1. DEFINITION

      a. Any *opacity* or *decreased clarity* of the lens or its capsule.

      b. Etiologies

        (1) Congenital

          (a) **Intrauterine rubella**.

          (b) *Herpes simplex*

          (c) *Herpes zoster*

          (d) Syphilis

          (e) Cytomegalic inclusion disease

        (2) Chromosomal disorders

          Down syndrome

        (3) Idiopathic or inherited

          (a) Aging

             A senile cataract is the most common cause of lens opacity

          (b) Metabolic

             Diabetes mellitus

          (c) Traumatic

             ▸ Blunt trauma

             ▸ Intraocular foreign body

             ▸ Radiation

(d) Drug-induced
The long-term use of systemic steroids.

2. DIAGNOSIS

Ophthalmoscopic and/or slit lamp examination reveals lens opacity or decreased clarity.

3. TREATMENT

a. Lenses to improve visual acuity.

b. Eventually, surgery is the definitive therapy.

VI. GLAUCOMA

A. *Primary Open-Angle Glaucoma*

1. DEFINITION

a. An *elevated intraocular pressure*, >22 mm Hg resulting from the ↓ aqueous outflow through the trabecular network.

b. There is gradual, painless *degeneration of the optic nerve* and loss of visual fields.

c. **The most common type of glaucoma.**

d. Visual loss begins at the periphery.

2. DIAGNOSIS

a. Increased intraocular pressure by tonometry

b. Visual field loss

c. Optic nerve changes

3. TREATMENT

a. Topical solutions

(1) Cholinergics to increase aqueous outflow

(a) Pilocarpine

(b) Carbachol

(c) Echothiophate

(2) Adrenergic agonists

Epinephrine dipivefrin

(3) Beta-adrenergic blocking agents to decrease aqueous formation.

(a) Timolol

(b) Levobunalol

(c) Betaxolol

b. Systemic carbonic anhydrase inhibitors to further decrease aqueous formation.

Acetazolamide

c. Failure of medical therapy

Laser trabeculoplasty or filtration surgery

B. *Secondary Open-Angle Glaucoma*
1. Etiologies
a. Malignancies
(1) Leukemia
(2) Neoplastic metastases
b. Intraocular inflammation
c. **Chronic use of ophthalmologic or systemic steroids**
C. *Primary Angle-Closure Glaucoma*
1. DEFINITION
a. An *elevated intraocular pressure*, >22 mm Hg resulting from the *obstruction* of aqueous outflow through the trabecular network *by the iris*.
b. **Acute onset of primary angle-closure glaucoma is ophthalmologic emergency.**
2. DIAGNOSIS
a. Pain
b. Tearing
c. Blurred vision
d. Nausea and vomiting
e. Mid-range to fixed pupil
f. Markedly increased intraocular pressures (40-80 mm Hg).
g. Corneal edema
h. Conjunctival hyperemia
3. TREATMENT
a. Rapid reduction of intraocular pressure
(1) Oral glycerine or sorbitol
(2) Intravenous mannitol
b. Early laser iridectomy.
D. *Secondary Angle-Closure Glaucoma*
1. Occurs from the formation of a neovascular network.
a. Etiologies
(1) Diabetic retinopathy
(2) Inflammatory synechiae

VII. **DISEASES OF THE RETINA**
A. *Hypertensive Retinopathy*
1. Grade I
Arteriole narrowing
2. Grade II
a. Arteriovenous nicking
b. Minimal exudates
c. Splinter hemorrhages

3. Grade III
   a. Retinal edema
   b. Exudates
   c. Hemorrhages
   d. Cotton-wool spots
4. Grade IV
   The above + papilledema
B. *Diabetic Retinopathy*
   1. DEFINITION
      a. Increased retinal blood flow followed by breakdown of the blood-retina barrier and movement of large molecules into the extracellular space of the retina causing macular edema.
         (1) Simple (Background) Retinopathy
             (a) Microaneurysms
             (b) Dot hemorrhages
             (c) Hard lipid exudates
             (d) Intraretinal microvascular abnormalities
         (2) Proliferative
             (a) There is retinal vessel growth *into* the vitreous, usually at the disk.
             (b) The vessels may bleed causing a vitreous hemorrhage.
   2. DIAGNOSIS
      Ophthalmoscopic or slit lamp examination
   3. TREATMENT
      Laser photocoagulation therapy

VIII. OCULAR TUMORS
A. *Retinoblastoma*
   1. DEFINITION
      a. A malignant tumor arising directly from the retina.
      b. The retinoblastoma is the most common malignant ocular tumor in children.
   2. DIAGNOSIS
      a. Absence of the "red" reflex
      b. Leukocoria
         Presence of the "white" pupil
      c. Strabismus
      d. Visual disturbance
      e. Erythema
      f. Pain
      g. Hyphema

3. TREATMENT
   a. Enucleation
   b. Radiation
   c. Chemotherapy
   d. Photocoagulation and cryotherapy may be effective on smaller lesions.
4. PROGNOSIS
   Poor

B. *Melanoma*
   1. DEFINITION
      a. Most common malignant intraocular tumor arises from the choroid *not* the retina.
      b. Presents in the 50-60s, silent until the growth impairs vision
   2. DIAGNOSIS
      Ophthalmoscopic or slit lamp examination
   3. TREATMENT
      a. Enucleation
      b. Local resection
      c. Photocoagulation
   4. PROGNOSIS
      a. 5-year survival
         (1) 50% if no metastasis at diagnosis
         (2) Poor if metastasis present

I. THE EAR
A. External Ear Infections
1. *Acute otitis externa*
a. DEFINITION
(1) "Swimmer's ear" An infection of the ear canal.
(2) Localized otitis externa
(a) Etiologies
  ‣ *Staphylococcus aureus*
  ‣ Group A streptococcus
(3) Diffuse otitis externa
(a) Etiologies
  ‣ *Pseudomonas aeruginosa*
  ‣ *Staphylococcus aureus*
(4) Necrotizing (Malignant) otitis externa
(a) This is a potentially life-threatening infection usually occurring in elderly diabetics.
(b) Invasion of the soft tissues may lead to osteomyelitis of the base of the skull and cranial nerve palsies
(c) Etiology
  Pseudomonas aeruginosa

b. DIAGNOSIS
(1) **Pain**
(2) **Pruritus**
(3) Discharge
(4) ± hearing loss
(5) Otoscopic exam
(a) Erythema
(b) Edema
(c) Exudate
(6) ± lymphadenopathy

c. TREATMENT
(1) Mild disease
(a) Clean the canal
(b) Topical antibiotic and/or steroid drops
(c) 2-5% acetic acid drops
(2) Severe infection
(a) A cotton wick is inserted into the canal so drops can penetrate.
(b) Appropriate systemic antibiotic dependent upon etiology
(3) Malignant (invasive) otitis externa
(a) Systemic antibiotic therapy
  ‣ Quinolones
  ‣ Anti-pseudomonal cephalosporins
  ‣ Anti-pseudomonal penicillins + aminoglycosides

(b) Debridement
2. *Otomycosis*
   a. DEFINITION
      (1) "Fungus or Jungle ear" A chronic fungal infection of the ear canal.
      (2) Etiologies
         (a) *Aspergillus niger*
         (b) *Candida albicans*
   b. DIAGNOSIS
      Otoscopic exam reveals whitish-grey, yellow or black exudate in the canal
   c. TREATMENT
      (1) Clean and debride
      (2) Acidify the canal
      (3) ± antibiotic drops
B. Middle Ear Disease
   1. *Acute Otitis Media*
      a. DEFINITION
         (1) A *bacterial* or *viral* infection of the middle ear.
         (2) A preceding viral URI produces eustachian tube dysfunction creating a partial vacuum in the middle ear. Serum moves into the middle ear to alleviate the vacuum and equalize the pressure, infection follows.
         (3) Classification
            (a) Acute otitis media → infection resolving within 3 weeks
            (b) Subacute otitis media → infection resolving in 3 weeks to 3 months
            (c) Chronic otitis media → infection lasting > 3 months
         (4) Most common etiologies
            (a) *Streptococcus pneumoniae*
            (b) *Hemophilus influenzae*
            (c) *Moraxella catarrhalis*
            (d) Gram-negative bacilli
               ≈ 20% of cases in infants less than six weeks old
            (e) Group A streptococci and *Staphylococcus aureus* are rare.
      b. DIAGNOSIS
         (1) Acute suppurative otitis media
            (a) The tympanic membrane is red, bulging and *immobile* by pneumatic otoscopy.
            (b) Often the light reflex is lost when the membrane bulges
            (c) ± fever
            (d) Pain
            (e) There may be *unilateral* hearing loss
      c. TREATMENT
         (1) **Aeration of the middle ear is essential in the treatment of otitis media.**

(2) Topical and/or systemic decongestants

(3) Antibiotic therapy

    (a) **Group A beta-hemolytic streptococci**
- Penicillin
- Erythromycin if penicillin allergic

    (b) *Hemophilus influenzae*
- Second or third generation cephalosporin
- Trimethoprim/sulfamethoxazole
- Amoxicillin/clavulanic acid
- Macrolides
  - Clarithromycin
  - Azithromycin
- Fluoroquinolones
  Never used in infants and children

    (c) *Moraxella catarrhalis*
- Second or third generation cephalosporin
- Trimethoprim/sulfamethoxazole
- Amoxicillin/clavulanic acid
- Macrolides
  - Clarithromycin
  - Azithromycin
- Fluoroquinolones
  Never used in infants and children

(4) Antibiotic prophylaxis for recurrent otitis media

(5) **Adequate treatment = 10 days to two weeks. Always recheck for resolution of infection.**

2. *Serous (Subacute) Otitis Media*

    a. DEFINITION

        (1) The *retention* of fluid in the middle ear.

        (2) The fluid is a *transudate*.

    b. DIAGNOSIS

        (1) Dull grey, amber or red TM

        (2) Bubbles or air-fluid levels

        (3) The tympanic membrane is retracted and *moves* to *negative* pressure by pneumatic otoscopy.

        (4) ↑ vascularity + thickening of the membrane = decreased translucency.

    c. TREATMENT

        (1) Decongestant/antihistamine preps.

        (2) Antibiotic therapy is added when *bacterial* URI is present.

        (3) ± glucocorticoids

        (4) Valsalva maneuver

(5) Myringotomy + placement of tympanotomy tube(s) is indicated when
    (a) Refractory infection
    (b) Inability to tolerate antibiotics
    (c) >3 episodes of otitis in 6 months
    (d) Persistent effusion with hearing loss >25 decibels
    (e) Infection despite antibiotic prophylaxis

3. *Chronic Otitis Media*
    a. DEFINITION
        (1) Hearing loss + tympanic membrane and ossicle damage + chronic otorrhea ± pain.
        (2) Tympanic membrane perforation is usually present.
        (3) Chronic infection occurs as water penetrates the middle ear via perforation.
        (4) Common etiologies
            (a) *Pseudomonas aeruginosa*
            (b) *Staphylococcus aureus*
            (c) *E coli*
            (d) *Proteus* sp.
        (5) Cholesteatoma
            (a) Epithelium of the tympanic membrane retracts into the mastoid air cells, enlarges, keratizes, and forms an epithelial inclusion cyst.
            (b) It is cured by excision
            (c) **It's the most common cause of mastoiditis.**
    b. DIAGNOSIS
        Thickening of TM + calcific white patches + perforation(s) + discharge.
    c. TREATMENT
        (1) Appropriate topical and systemic antibiotics to clear infection
        (2) Surgical correction of the defect in the tympanic membrane

4. Complications of Otitis Media.
    a. Hearing loss
    b. Labyrinthritis
    c. Meningitis
    d. Extradural abscess
    e. Subdural empyema
    f. Otogenic abscess
    g. Lateral sinus thrombophlebitis

C. Tumors
    1. Benign
        a. *Exostosis*
            (1) **The most common tumor of the auditory canal.**

(2) Composed of dense compact bone, surgical removal if they become symptomatic by causing obstruction and secondary infection.

b. *Chemodectoma (Glomus tumor)*

(1) Arising from glomus bodies, they produce *pulsating tinnitus* followed by *hearing loss* and finally invasion of the TM. It may involve cranial nerves.

(2) A dark blue-to-purple mass by otoscopic exam.

(3) **Don't biopsy- It's a very vascular tumor.**

(4) Surgical removal is the treatment of choice.

c. *Acoustic neuroma*

(1) "Schwannoma" is composed of myelin-forming schwann cells
8% of all brain tumors and 80% of all posterior fossa tumors.

(2) Unilateral tinnitus + gradual onset of unilateral sensoneural hearing loss, think acoustic neuroma.

(3) 10% present with episodic vertigo.

(4) The majority arise from the vestibular division of the eighth cranial nerve.

(5) CT scan or MRI very helpful in diagnosis.

(6) Surgery is the treatment of choice.

2. Malignant

a. *Squamous cell carcinoma*

(1) **The most common tumor.**

(2) Surgical resection is the treatment of choice.

(3) Prognosis

(a) Guarded to poor

(b) Dependent upon the amount of extension into the temporal and petrous bones.

D. *Vertigo*

1. **Dizziness is a sensation of altered orientation in space.**

2. **Vertigo is a type of dizziness caused by disease of the vestibular system.**

3. The lesion may be central
The eighth cranial nerve and central nervous system

4. The lesion may be peripheral
Pathology involving the inner ear

5. Common causes of episodic vertigo resulting from inner ear pathology

a. *Benign Paroxysmal Positional Vertigo*

(1) DEFINITION

(a) A *change of position* triggers the dizziness.

(b) The surrounding environment spins for 10-20 seconds then resolves until the patient initiates a similar movement.

(2) DIAGNOSIS

(a) Physical examination is usually normal

(b) A diagnosis of exclusion.

(c) You must rule out organic disease involving the CNS or the ears *before* the diagnosis is made.

(3) TREATMENT

    (a) Supportive therapy

    (b) A self-limiting condition that usually resolves in four to six weeks.

b. *Meniere's Disease*

  (1) DEFINITION

    (a) **Recurrent episodic vertigo + tinnitus + unilateral hearing loss + pressure or fullness in the affected ear.**

    (b) Etiology unknown.

    (c) 30-40% have bilateral disease

    (d) No neurologic deficits

    (e) Dizziness can last a few minutes to a few hours. Severe cases can last for days.

  (2) TREATMENT

    (a) Dietary modification

- Low salt diet
- Low fat diet
- Decrease or discontinue caffeine
- Decrease or discontinue alcohol
- Decrease or discontinue chocolate
- Stop smoking

    (b) Vestibular suppressants and sedatives

- IV or PO diazepam
- Transdermal scopolamine
- Meclizine

    (c) Antiemetics

    (d) Diuretics

    (e) Surgery (10-20% of patients)

- Decompression of endolymph sac works >70% of the time to relieve vertigo.
- Failure of the endolymphatic sac-enhancement surgery
  - Vestibular neurectomy
  - Labyrinthectomy
- No procedure corrects the hearing loss.

II. SINUS

A. *Sinusitis*

  1. DEFINITION

    a. An inflammation of the mucosa of the paranasal sinuses.

b. Etiologies
  (1) Acute viral
    (a) Rhinovirus
    (b) Adenovirus
    (c) Influenza
    (d) Parainfluenza
  (2) Acute bacterial
    (a) *Streptococcus pneumoniae*
    (b) *Hemophilis influenzae*
    (c) *Moraxella catarrhalis*
    (d) *Streptococcus pyogenes*
  (3) Chronic
    (a) The organisms listed above causing acute sinusitis
    (b) *Staphylococcus aureus*
    (c) Anaerobes

2. DIAGNOSIS
  a. History and physical
    (1) Pressure and congestion
    (2) Nasal discharge
    (3) Headache
    (4) Fatigue
    (5) Pain over cheeks and upper teeth, eyebrows or behind eyes
    (6) Postnasal discharge
    (7) Fever
  b. Laboratory
    (1) Leukocytosis in acute bacterial sinusitis.
    (2) Cultures may identify bacterial organisms
    (3) X-rays are not needed for acute sinusitis but for evaluation of chronic sinusitis or possible complications
      (a) Plain films of the sinuses
      (b) CT
      (c) MRI
        To evaluate possible tumor or fungal infection

3. TREATMENT
  a. **Promote adequate drainage**
    Topical and/or systemic decongestants
  b. Antihistamines are not indicated unless there is underlying allergy because they thicken secretions.
  c. Antibiotic therapy
    (1) **Group A beta-hemolytic streptococci**
      (a) Penicillin

(b) Erythromycin if penicillin allergic
(2) *Hemophilus influenzae*
 (a) Second or third generation cephalosporin
 (b) Trimethoprim/sulfamethoxazole
 (c) Amoxicillin/clavulanic acid
 (d) Macrolides
  ‣ Clarithromycin
  ‣ Azithromycin
 (e) Fluoroquinolones
  Never used in infants and children
(3) *Moraxella catarrhalis*
 (a) Second or third generation cephalosporin
 (b) Trimethoprim/sulfamethoxazole
 (c) Amoxicillin/clavulanic acid
 (d) Macrolides
  ‣ Clarithromycin
  ‣ Azithromycin
 (e) Fluoroquinolones
  Never used in infants and children
d. **Adequate therapy = 10-14 days. Always recheck for resolution of infection.**
e. Refractory cases of chronic sinusitis
 (1) Surgery
 (2) Allergy and/or immunologic consultation
4. COMPLICATIONS
 a. Orbital cellulitis
 b. Meningitis
 c. Extradural abscess
 d. Subdural abscess
 e. Brain abscess
 f. Osteomyelitis

III. NOSE
A. *Allergic Rhinitis*
 1. DEFINITION
  a. "Hay fever"
  b. An inflammatory condition of the nose characterized by rhinorrhea, congestion, and sneezing.
  c. It may be associated with conjunctival itching and tearing.
   (1) *Seasonal allergic rhinitis*
    Molds, grasses, trees and pollen.

            (2) *Perennial allergic rhinitis*

                Dust, dander, cigarette smoke and foods.

      d. **An IgE-dependent triggering of mast cells in sensitized individuals**.

2. DIAGNOSIS

    a. Pale, swollen nasal mucosa associated with a thin clear, watery discharge.

    b. Conjunctiva may be injected.

    c. Laboratory

        (1) CBC

            Normal white cell count, ↑ eosinophils

        (2) ↑ IgE levels

        (3) Skin and RAST testing

3. TREATMENT

    a. Decreasing exposure to allergens

    b. Antihistamines and/or decongestants

    c. Intranasal steroids

    d. Intranasal cromolyn

    e. Systemic steroids in severe cases

    f. Hyposensitization

    g. **Avoid excessive use of topical decongestants because of rebound congestion.**

B. *Nasal Polyposis*

  1. DEFINITION

    a. Arising from the nasal or sinus mucosa, polyps are soft, lobulated masses that may cause partial or complete nasal obstruction.

    b. Associated with

        (1) Chronic allergic rhinitis

        (2) Cystic fibrosis

        (3) Aspirin-induced asthma

        (4) Chronic sinusitis

  2. DIAGNOSIS

    The lesions are painless, not fixed to the underlying tissues and don't hemorrhage.

  3. TREATMENT

    a. Medical

        Antihistamines and/or decongestants, topical steroids.

    b. Surgical

        Polypectomy

D. *Epistaxis*

  1. DEFINITION

    "A nosebleed"

  2. DIAGNOSIS

    a. Most cases are *idiopathic* but don't forget about

        (1) Coagulopathies

(2) Trauma

(3) Neoplasms

(4) Infection

(5) Hypertension

(6) Vascular abnormalities

3. TREATMENT

a. Anterior bleed

(1) Manual pressure

(2) Cautery

(3) Nasal packing

b. Posterior bleed

Balloon systems for direct compression

c. Intractable bleed

Arterial ligation

E. TUMORS

1. **Tumors of the nose and paranasal sinuses are uncommon**

2. Benign tumors

Papilloma and *Osteoma* are excised if there is obstruction.

3. Malignant tumors

a. *Squamous cell carcinoma*

(1) **The most common malignancy**

(2) Even with surgery + radiation therapy, the prognosis is poor

IV. ORAL CAVITY

A. Lips and Mouth

1. Infections

a. *Acute necrotizing ulcerative gingivitis*

(1) DEFINITION

"Trench Mouth" An acute fusospirochetal infection of the gingiva.

(2) DIAGNOSIS

(a) The *"Three B's"* Bad breath, bad taste and bleeding of the gingiva.

(b) "Punched out" lesions on interdental papillae and mucous membranes covered with a grayish necrotic membrane.

(3) TREATMENT

(a) Good oral hygiene

(b) Penicillin

2. Tumors

a. Benign

(1) *Fibromas, Hemangiomas, and Papillomas*

(a) They can occur anywhere in the oral cavity.

(b) If symptomatic they can be removed surgically.

(2) *Exostoses*

    (a) **Torus Palatinus**

        ‣ A bony growth on the hard palate.

        ‣ Surgery only if a prosthetic device is needed.

b. Malignant

    (1) *Squamous cell carcinoma*

        (a) Usually involves the tongue and floor of mouth.

        (b) **95% of oral tumors.**

        (c) TREATMENT

            Surgery and radiation therapy.

        (d) PROGNOSIS

            Five-year survival ≈30%.

B. SALIVARY GLANDS

1. *Sialadenitis*

    a. DEFINITION

        (1) An inflammation or infection of the salivary gland or excretory duct.

        (2) Etiologies

            (a) Bacteria from the oral cavity most common.

            (b) Mumps

    b. DIAGNOSIS

        (1) A swollen, tender salivary gland

        (2) ± purulent discharge from the duct

    c. TREATMENT

        (1) Penicillin

        (2) Erythromycin

2. *Sialolithiasis*

    a. DEFINITION

        (1) The presence of calculi *within* the ducts of any of the major salivary glands.

        (2) Calculi are secondary to

            (a) Trauma

            (b) Inflammation

            (c) Chronic diseases which cause stasis of saliva or alter its secretion.

        (3) 90% of occurrences are in the submandibular glands.

    b. DIAGNOSIS

        (1) Pain and swelling of the salivary gland upon eating

        (2) Sialogram is usually diagnostic since 80% of calculi are radiopaque.

    c. TREATMENT

        Removal of the stone by massage and/or surgery.

3. Tumors

    a. Benign

        (1) **Pleomorphic adenoma**
           (a) The most common tumor.
           (b) Benign but will reoccur unless completely removed
        (2) Monomorphic Adenoma
        (3) Warthin's Tumor
    b. Malignant
        (1) Mucoepidermoid carcinoma
        (2) Adenoid cystic carcinoma
        (3) Adenocarcinoma
    c. DIAGNOSIS
        (1) Slow growing, *painless* mass
        (2) Palpation reveals enlargement
        (3) CT or MRI diagnostic
    d. TREATMENT
      Surgery
    e. PROGNOSIS
        (1) Mucoepidermoid carcinoma
           (a) 5-year survival
               Dependent upon the grade of the tumor, $\approx$ 50-90%
        (2) Adenoid cystic carcinoma
           (a) 5-year survival...........$\approx$65%
           (b) 20-year survival.........$\approx$15%
C. TEMPOROMANDIBULAR DISEASE
  1. *Temporomandibular disorders*
    a. DEFINITION
        (1) An inflammation of the temporomandibular joint or the major and minor muscles of mastication.
        (2) Etiologies
           (a) Malocclusion
           (b) Displacement of the condylar head
           (c) Bruxism
           (d) Trauma
           (e) Acute synovitis
           (f) Arthritis
    b. DIAGNOSIS
        (1) Pain upon opening and closing the mouth, with or without deviation of the jaw.
        (2) Pain to palpation of the joint.
        (3) Arthroscopy or CT helpful.
    c. TREATMENT
        (1) NSAIDs

(2) Anxiolytics and/or antidepressants

(3) Analgesics

(4) Orthodontic appliance

(5) Muscle relaxants

(6) Psychotherapy

(7) Surgery

V. THROAT
A. INFECTIONS
1. *Acute Pharyngitis*
a. DEFINITION
(1) "A sore throat"

(2) An inflammation of the mucous membranes of the throat most often caused by an infectious agent.

(3) **One third of cases of pharyngitis is secondary to Group A beta-hemolytic streptococci.**

(4) One third of cases of pharyngitis have no detectable infectious etiology

(5) Viral and bacterial pharyngitis may be indistinguishable on clinical exam.

(6) Etiologies
   (a) Bacterial
   - **Group A beta-hemolytic streptococci**
   - *Hemophilus influenzae*
   - *Moraxella catarrhalis*

   (b) Less frequent bacterial etiologies
   - *Mycoplasma pneumoniae*
   - *Arcanebacterium hemolyticum*
   - *Neisseria gonorrhoeae*
   - *Groups C and G streptococci*
   - *Chlamydia pneumoniae*
   - *Corynebacterium diphtheriae*

   (c) Viral
   - Rhinovirus
   - Adenovirus
   - Parainfluenza
   - Epstein-Barr

b. DIAGNOSIS
(1) Pharyngeal erythema ± exudates

(2) Dysphagia

(3) ± palatal petechiae

(4) Cervical adenopathy

(5) Tonsillar enlargement

(6) Fever, chills and headache

(7) ± nausea

(8) Laboratory

   (a) CBC

   Leukocytosis in bacterial pharyngitis.

   (b) Rapid antigen detection

   A negative test doesn't exclude the possibility of streptococcal infection

   (c) Throat cultures

   Neisseria gonorrhoeae, Corynebacterium diphtheriae and *Arcanebacterium hemolyticum* require special cultures

   (d) Heterophil agglutinin

   Detection of the Epstein-Barr virus and the diagnosis of infectious mononucleosis

c. TREATMENT

   (1) The majority of pharyngitis is self-limiting and doesn't require antibiotics

   (2) **Group A beta-hemolytic streptococci**

   (a) Penicillin

   (b) Erythromycin if penicillin allergic

   (3) *Hemophilus influenzae*

   (a) Second or third generation cephalosporin

   (b) Trimethoprim/sulfamethoxazole

   (c) Amoxicillin/clavulanic acid

   (d) Macrolides

   ▸ Clarithromycin

   ▸ Azithromycin

   (e) Fluoroquinolones

   (4) *Moraxella catarrhalis*

   (a) Second or third generation cephalosporin

   (b) Trimethoprim/sulfamethoxazole

   (c) Amoxicillin/clavulanic acid

   (d) Macrolides

   ▸ Clarithromycin

   ▸ Azithromycin

   (e) Fluoroquinolones

   (5) **Adequate treatment = 10 days. Always recheck for resolution of infection.**

2. *Peritonsillar Abscess*

   a. DEFINITION

   (1) An abscess in the peritonsillar space that occurs as a sequelae to acute tonsillitis or tonsillopharyngitis.

(2) Etiology

Most often beta-hemolytic streptococci

b. DIAGNOSIS

(1) Fever

(2) Severe pain

(3) Dysphagia

(4) A swollen tonsil with indurated, erythematous peritonsillar tissues.

(5) Laboratory

(a) Leukocytosis

(b) Throat culture

(c) Rapid Strep test

c. TREATMENT

(1) Children

Hospitalize, IV antibiotics usually a penicillin for 10 to 14 days

(2) Adults

(a) Outpatient unless there is dehydration or they become toxic

(b) Abscess may have to be incised and drained

(c) Antibiotics

Usually a penicillin or a cephalosporin, 10 to 14 days

VI. LARYNX

A. INFECTIONS

1. *Acute epiglottitis*

a. DEFINITION

(1) A potentially fatal infection of the supraglottic tissues.

(2) **It is a rapidly progressive cellulitis of the epiglottis and the supraglottic tissues.**

(3) Etiologies

(a) Children

Hemophilus influenzae type b.

(b) Adults

‣ Group A, beta-hemolytic streptococci.

‣ *Streptococcus pneumoniae*

‣ *Hemophilus influenzae*

b. DIAGNOSIS

(1) Rapid onset of fever

(2) Severe pharyngitis

(3) Respiratory distress associated with difficulty swallowing and drooling

(4) **Don't ever stick a tongue depressor in a child's mouth if you suspect epiglottitis. It could trigger complete airway obstruction.**

(5) Laboratory

    (a) Leukocytosis

    (b) Cultures

        ▸ Throat

        ▸ Blood

    (c) Lateral X-ray of the neck

        "Thumb sign" = a thumb-shaped epiglottis

c. TREATMENT

    (1) Keep the patient calm.

    (2) Aggressive management of this infection is required

        (a) Antibiotics

            Usually with a third generation cephalosporin

        (b) *Controlled* intubation by an Anesthesiologist or Otorhino-laryngologist.

        (c) If intubation fails, then perform a tracheostomy

    (3) Racemic epinephrine and systemic steroids are contraindicated.

2. *Laryngotracheobronchitis*

    a. DEFINITION

        (1) "Croup" A respiratory infection in children causing laryngeal edema.

        (2) Etiology

            (a) Usually viral

                ▸ Parainfluenza

                ▸ Influenza A

                ▸ Respiratory syncytial virus

    b. DIAGNOSIS

        (1) Usually follows a URI with rapid development of

            (a) Fever

            (b) Hoarseness

            (c) Barking cough

        (2) Lateral X-ray of the neck

            Subglottic narrowing

        (3) There's respiratory distress manifest by inspiratory stridor and tachypnea

        (4) Symptoms are worse at night

    c. TREATMENT

        (1) Humidification

        (2) Hospitalization if there is significant respiratory distress

            ▸ Racemic epinephrine + saline nebulized

            ▸ Systemic steroids may be indicated.

3. *Acute Laryngitis*

    a. DEFINITION

        (1) An acute inflammation of the laryngeal mucosa.

(2) Etiologies

    (a) **Viral**

        Rhinovirus

    (b) Bacterial

        ‣ *Moraxella catarrhalis*

        ‣ *Hemophilus influenzae*

        ‣ *Streptococcus* spp.

b. DIAGNOSIS

    (1) Hoarseness ± URI.

    (2) Leukocytosis with bacterial URI.

c. TREATMENT

    (1) Voice rest

    (2) Decongestants

    (3) The majority of cases are self-limiting and doesn't require antibiotic therapy

    (4) If the laryngitis doesn't resolve in a couple of days think primary or secondary bacterial infection

    (5) Antibiotic therapy

        See treatment of pharyngitis V.A.1.c.

    (6) **Hoarseness > two weeks = laryngeal pathology ⇢ refer to an ENT.**

4. *Chronic Laryngitis*

    a. DEFINITION

        (1) A chronic inflammation of the laryngeal mucosal tissues.

        (2) Etiologies

            (a) Allergies and irritants

            (b) Smoking

            (c) ETOH

            (d) Voice abuse

            (e) Gastroesophageal reflux

            (f) Respiratory infections ± cough

    b. DIAGNOSIS

        Laryngoscopy

    c. TREATMENT

        (1) Treat the underlying etiology

        (2) Voice rest.

        (3) Laryngoscopy, if vocal cords are hyperplastic or leukoplakia is present, strip the membranes and biopsy any areas of leukoplakia.

B. LARYNGEAL NEOPLASMS

    1. Benign

        a. *Polyps*

            (1) Chronic irritation + a vocal cord = edema of the cord.

            (2) Hoarseness follows, often with the formation of a polyp.

            (3) Treatment is surgical

      b. *Papillomata*

            (1) A common laryngeal neoplasm of viral etiology

            (2) Treatment is surgical

2. Malignant

    a. DEFINITION

            (1) **Squamous cell carcinoma**

                  >90% of malignant laryngeal tumors

    b. DIAGNOSIS

        Chronic hoarseness followed by laryngoscopy and biopsy

    c. TREATMENT

        Surgery and/or radiation therapy

    d. PROGNOSIS

            (1) 5-year survival

                (a) >80% for lesions on the true cords.

                (b) >50% for lesions above the true cords.

I. INFECTIONS

A. *Acute Bronchitis*

   1. DEFINITION

      a. An infection of the trachea, bronchi and/or bronchioles *usually* caused by a *viral* infection.

      b. **Do not confuse this illness with an acute exacerbation of chronic bronchitis the etiology of which is usually bacterial.**

      c. Etiologies

         (1) Viral

            (a) Rhinovirus

            (b) Adenovirus

            (c) Influenza A and B

            (d) Parainfluenza.

         (2) Bacterial

            (a) *Streptococcal pneumoniae*

            (b) *Hemophilus influenzae*

            (c) *Moraxella catarrhalis*

         (3) Atypicals

            (a) *Mycoplasma pneumoniae*

            (b) *Chlamydia pneumoniae*

   2. DIAGNOSIS

      a. URI + cough which becomes productive

      b. Fever, myalgias, fatigue

      c. Occasional dyspnea

      d. Crackles and rhonchi may be present

      e. Laboratory

         (1) If bacterial etiology is considered, leukocytosis

         (2) Gram stain of sputum will help with diagnosis

   3. TREATMENT

      a. Supportive therapy for viral illnesses

      b. For treatment of specific bacteria and atypicals

B. Community-Acquired Pneumonia (CAP)

   1. *Streptococcus pneumoniae*

      a. DEFINITION

         (1) An acute infection of the lung parenchyma caused by *Streptococcus pneumoniae*.

         (2) *Streptococcus pneumoniae* is also called pneumococcus.

         (3) It is the most common etiology of community-acquired pneumonia in all age groups.

      b. DIAGNOSIS

         (1) Fever, chills, headache

         (2) Nausea and vomiting

         (3) Chest pain

       (4) Purulent or rust-colored sputum

       (5) Blood-tinged sputum, classically with dense lobar consolidation.

       (6) Decreased breath sounds

       (7) Dyspnea

       (8) Crackles and/or rhonchi

       (9) Tachypnea

       (10) Laboratory

            (a) *Gram stain*

                Gram + encapsulated, elongated, paired cocci.

            (b) + blood cultures about a third of the time.

            (c) Leukocytosis with left shift

            (d) Bacteremia <33% of the time.

            (e) Chest X-ray

                Lobar consolidation or patchy bronchopneumonia

c. TREATMENT

       (1) Early antibiotic therapy improves outcome.

       (2) Penicillins are the drug of choice

            (a) With an increasing incidence of pneumococcal resistance to peni-cillins some advocate the use of cephalosporins or macrolides for *empirical* treatment of choice.

            (b) Once sensitivities are determined and no resistance is noted, peni-cillin is usually adequate.

       (3) Pneumococcal vaccine for prophylaxis is available

2. *Hemophilus influenzae*

  a. DEFINITION

        An acute infection of the lung parenchyma caused by *Hemophilus influenzae*.

  b. DIAGNOSIS

       (1) Second only to *Streptococcus pneumoniae* as the etiology of CAP.

       (2) Signs and symptoms and laboratory similar to *Streptococcus pneumoniae*.

       (3) *Gram stain*

              Pleomorphic gram-negative rods

  c. TREATMENT

       (1) Second or third generation cephalosporins

       (2) Amoxicillin-clavulanic acid

       (3) Trimethoprim-sulfamethoxazole

       (4) Macrolides

            ▸ Clarithromycin

            ▸ Azithromycin

       (5) Avoid penicillins, tetracyclines, and first generation cephalosporins because of resistance

3. *Moraxella catarrhalis*
    a. DEFINITION
        An acute infection of the lung parenchyma caused by *Moraxella catarrhalis*
    b. DIAGNOSIS
        (1) <5% of all pneumonias, more commonly observed in patients with COPD
        (2) Chest X-ray
            Patchy bronchopulmonary infiltrate
        (3) Lobar consolidation is rare
        (4) *Gram stain*
            Kidney bean-shaped gram-negative diplococci
    c. TREATMENT
        (1) Second or third generation cephalosporins
        (2) Amoxicillin-Clavulanic acid
        (3) Quinolones
        (4) Macrolides
            ▸ Clarithromycin
            ▸ Azithromycin
        (5) Trimethoprim-sulfamethoxazole
        (6) Tetracycline
        (7) **Avoid penicillins, because of resistance.**

4. *Staphylococcal* pneumonia
    a. DEFINITION
        Acute infection of the lung parenchyma caused by *Staphylococcus aureus*
        or *Staphylococcus epidermidis.*
    b. DIAGNOSIS
        (1) <10% of all community-acquired pneumonias
        (2) **Occurs in debilitated or chronically ill patients**
        (3) Signs and symptoms and laboratory similar to streptococcal pneumonia
        (4) ↑ incidence of tissue necrosis, cavitation and empyema
        (5) Chest X-ray
            ▸ **Bilateral consolidation ≈60% of the time**
            ▸ Effusion or empyema ≈50% of the time
        (6) *Gram stain*
            Clumps (grape-like clusters) of gram + cocci
    c. TREATMENT
        (1) Semisynthetic penicillins
        (2) Cephalosporins
        (3) Trimethoprim-sulfamethoxazole
        (4) Quinolones
        (5) Clindamycin
        (6) **Avoid penicillin, macrolides, tetracycline because of resistance**

5. *Gram-negative bacilli*
   a. DEFINITION
      (1) An acute infection of the lung parenchyma caused by gram-negative bacilli.
      (2) Etiologies
         (a) *Klebsiella pneumoniae*
         (b) *E coli*
         (c) *Enterobacter* sp.
         (d) *Pseudomonas aeruginosa*
   b. DIAGNOSIS
      (1) <15% of all community-acquired pneumonia
      (2) **Usually occurs in a debilitated or chronically ill patient**
      (3) Virulent infections with a host of complications
         (a) Necrosis
         (b) Cavitation
         (c) Empyema
      (4) Signs and symptoms of streptococcal pneumonia
      (5) *Gram stain*
        Gram-negative bacilli
   c. TREATMENT
      Third generation cephalosporin ± aminoglycoside
6. *Aspiration pneumonia*
   a. DEFINITION
      (1) An acute infection of the lung parenchyma caused by *aspiration* of anaerobic oropharyngeal bacteria.
      (2) Many times there is a *mixed flora* of anaerobes and aerobic bacteria.
      (3) Anaerobic etiologies
         (a) *Bacteroides fragilis*
         (b) *Fusobacterium* sp.
         (c) *Peptostreptococcus*
         (d) Microaerophilic streptococci
         (e) Peptococci
      (4) Aerobic etiologies
         (a) *Klebsiella pneumoniae*
         (b) *E coli*
         (c) *Enterobacter* sp.
         (d) *Pseudomonas aeruginosa*
   b. DIAGNOSIS
      (1) <15% of all community-acquired pneumonia
      (2) **It is most commonly observed in patients with neurologic disease or impairment**
      (3) Patients with esophageal dysfunction are also predisposed

(4) This pneumonia is *necrotizing*.

(5) Signs and symptoms

    (a) Low-grade fever

    (b) Weight loss

    (c) Productive cough producing foul smelling sputum

(6) Laboratory

    (a) CBC

        Leukocytosis

    (b) Chest X-ray

        ▸ Infiltrate most often involves the dependent lobes of the lungs

        ▸ Cavitation can occur with ± air-fluid levels

(7) Gram stain and cultures are not reliable.

c. TREATMENT

(1) Clindamycin

(2) Penicillin + metronidazole

(3) If there is risk of aerobic gram-negative bacilli *empirical* therapy pending culture and sensitivities may also include

    (a) Third generation cephalosporin with anaerobic coverage

    (b) Extended spectrum penicillin + an aminoglycoside

7. Atypical Pneumonias

  a. *Mycoplasma* pneumonia

    (1) DEFINITION

        An *interstitial* infection of the lung parenchyma by *Mycoplasma pneumoniae*, an organism that *lacks* a cell wall.

    (2) DIAGNOSIS

        (a) More common in children and young adults

        (b) Signs and symptoms

            ▸ *Gradual* onset of fatigue, fever, headache

            ▸ Chronic *non-productive* cough

        (c) Flu-like symptoms

            URI initially with <10% developing pneumonia

        (d) Laboratory

            ▸ CBC

                Leukocytosis ≈25% of the time

            ▸ Chest X-ray

                ▸ "Looks worse than the patient"

                ▸ Two presentations

                    • Lobar or segmental consolidation ± atelectasis

                    • Bilateral diffuse reticulonodular pattern

            ▸ Cultures

            ▸ Monoclonal antibody assay

(e) **Elevated cold agglutinins are nonspecific**

(3) TREATMENT

 (a) Macrolides

  ▸ Erythromycin

  ▸ Clarithromycin

  ▸ Azithromycin

 (b) Doxycycline or tetracycline

b. *Chlamydia* pneumonia

 (1) DEFINITION

  An acute infection of the lung parenchyma caused by the obligate intra-cellular gram-negative bacterium by *Chlamydia pneumoniae*.

 (2) DIAGNOSIS

  (a) More common in young adults

  (b) Clinical picture similar to *Mycoplasma* pneumonia.

  (c) History and physical

   ▸ Severe sore throat ± hoarseness one week before pneumonia

   ▸ Nonproductive cough

   ▸ ± crackles

  (d) Laboratory

   ▸ Chest X-ray

    Single segmental infiltrate

   ▸ Serologies used for diagnosis

 (3) TREATMENT

  (a) Tetracycline or Doxycycline

  (b) Macrolides

c. *Legionella pneumophilia*

 (1) DEFINITION

  An acute infection of the lung parenchyma caused by the aerobic gram-negative rod *Legionella pneumophilia*.

 (2) DIAGNOSIS

  (a) This is a virulent organism, causing more severe disease than the other atypicals.

  (b) **Think aerosolization of contaminated water**

  (c) **Think pneumonia following travel**

  (d) Signs and symptoms

   ▸ Fever ± chills

   ▸ Myalgia

   ▸ Headache

   ▸ Cough

   ▸ Pleuritic chest pain

   ▸ Abdominal pain

              ▸ Diarrhea
          (e) **Extrapulmonary involvement**
              ▸ Neurologic
                  • Encephalitis
                  • Cerebellar ataxia
              ▸ Gastrointestinal
                 Hepatitis
              ▸ Cardiovascular
                  • Pericarditis
                  • Myocarditis
              ▸ Kidney
                 Glomerulonephritis
          (f) Laboratory
              ▸ Normal to ↑ WBC count
              ▸ Marked ↑ ESR
              ▸↑ liver function studies
              ▸Chest X-ray
                 Unilateral lung infiltrates that progress bilaterally
              ▸ Florescent antibody studies of sputum
              ▸ **Radioimmunoassay**
                 Detects antigen in the urine
              ▸ **It cannot be seen on routine Gram stain.**
      (3) TREATMENT
          (a) Erythromycin ± rifampin for severe disease.
          (b) Clarithromycin
          (c) Doxycycline
          (d) Ciprofloxacin
          (e) Trimethoprim-sulfamethoxazole ± rifampin
C. Hospital-Acquired Pneumonia (Nosocomial)
    1. DEFINITION
        a. Pneumonia which occurs during hospitalization is a complication .5-1% of the time.
        b. **The mortality is 30-50%.**
        c. Etiologies
           (1) Gram-negative bacilli
               (a) ***Pseudomonas* sp.**
              (b) *Klebsiella* sp.
              (c) *E coli*
              (d) *Enterobacter* sp.
              (e) *Proteus* sp.
          (2) *Staphylococcus aureus*
          (3) *Streptococcus* spp.

2. DIAGNOSIS
    a. Fever
    b. Purulent sputum
    c. Tachypnea
    d. Leukocytosis
    e. New or progressive infiltrate
    f. ↑ in alveolar-arterial pO_2 gradient
    g. Oliguria
    h. Change in mental status

3. TREATMENT
    a. A second or third generation cephalosporin + an aminoglycoside
    b. An antipseudomonal penicillin ± vancomycin

D. *Viral Pneumonia*
  1. DEFINITION
    a. An acute viral infection of the lung parenchyma by:
      (1) Influenza A and B
      (2) Respiratory syncytial virus
      (3) Adenovirus
      (4) Rubeola
      (5) *Herpes simplex*
      (6) Varicella
      (7) CMV (Cytomegalovirus) in an immunocompromised host.

  2. DIAGNOSIS
    a. History and physical
      (1) Fever and chills
      (2) Headache
      (3) Cough
      (4) Dyspnea
      (5) Crackles and rhonchi
    b. Laboratory
      (1) **Gram stain is negative**
      (2) CBC
          WBC normal or slightly leukopenic
      (3) Chest X-ray
          "Looks worse than the patient"

  3. TREATMENT
    a. Influenza A
      (1) Amantadine
      (2) Rimantadine

       b. Respiratory syncytial virus
          (1) Aerosolized ribavirin
             (a) Underlying pulmonary or cardiac disease
             (b) Immunologic disease
             (c) Infants with severe disease
       c. *Herpes simplex* or Varicella
          Acyclovir
       d. CMV
          (1) Ganciclovir
          (2) Foscarnet
       e. **There is a risk of secondary bacterial infection.**
  E. Criteria for hospitalization of patients with pneumonia
     1. "Vitals"
       a. Tachypnea > 30 breaths/minute
       b. Tachycardia > 140 beats/minute
       c. Hypotension < 90 mm Hg systolic
       d. Hypoxemia
     2. Age
       > 65 years of age
     3. Sensorium
       Acute change in mental status
     4. Etiology of pneumonia
       a. Gram-negative bacilli
       b. *Staphylococcus aureus*
       c. Anaerobes
     5. Underlying chronic illness
     6. Failure of outpatient therapy
     7. Leukopenia
       WBC < 5000/microliter
     8. Extrapulmonary complications
     9. Inability to take oral medication
 F. *Lung Abscess*
     1. DEFINITION
       a. A localized cavity within the lung parenchyma filled with pus.
       b. The pus is a product of necrosis of the lung tissue.
       c. The cavity is surrounded by infection
       d. Etiologies
          (1) Infectious
             (a) Suppurative pneumonia
             (b) Tuberculosis
             (c) Mycoses

(2) Aspiration of foreign body

(3) Pulmonary infarction

(4) Malignancy

2. DIAGNOSIS

    a. Fever, night sweats, chills

    b. Cough with ↑ production of putrid sputum

    c. Dyspnea

    d. Fatigue

    e. Weight loss

    f. Chest pain

    g. Hemoptysis

    h. Laboratory

        (1) *Chest X-ray*

            A solitary cavitary lesion with air fluid level

        (2) CBC

            Leukocytosis

        (3) Bronchoscopy

        (4) Tissue and/or sputum stains

            (a) Gram stain

            (b) Mycobacterial

            (c) Fungal stains

3. TREATMENT

    a. Antibiotics appropriate to culture and sensitivity

    b. Surgery

        (1) To remove foreign body

        (2) Treatment of malignancy

G. *Tuberculosis*

1. DEFINITION

    a. Pulmonary tuberculosis is a mycobacterial infection of the lung parenchyma.

    b. Etiologies

        (1) *Mycobacterium tuberculosis*

        (2) *Mycobacterium bovis*

        (3) *Mycobacterium africanum*

    c. Disseminated disease can occur involving the bones, kidneys and CNS.

2. DIAGNOSIS

    a. Fatigue

    b. Weight loss

    c. Cough

    d. ↑ sputum

    e. Hemoptysis

    f. Dyspnea

g. Chest pain

h. Laboratory

    (1) + **Acid-fast stain of sputum, body fluid or biopsied tissues.**

    (2) + PPD

    (3) **Chest X-ray**

        (a) ± effusion with primary disease.

        (b) Hilar adenopathy

        (c) Cavitary lesions upper lobes.

        (d) Ghon Complex

            A healed primary lesion with calcified hilar node and peripheral lesion

    (4) Florescent staining and DNA probes for rapid diagnosis.

3. TREATMENT

    a. Upon presumptive diagnosis of pulmonary TB immediate isolation and therapy

    b. Always check drug susceptibility when samples are cultured.

    c. ↑ resistance to medication

        (1) Multidrug-resistant tuberculosis

            (a) Organisms resistant to isoniazid and/or rifampin

            (b) HIV-positive patients are at ↑ risk for infection

    d. Antibiotic therapy

        (1) Isoniazid

        (2) Rifampin

        (3) Pyrazinamide

        (4) Ethambutol

        (5) Streptomycin

II. **PLEURAL EFFUSION**

A. DEFINITION

    1. An accumulation of fluid in the pleural space.

    2. Etiologies

        a. Transudates

            (1) CHF

            (2) Pneumonia

            (3) Hypoalbuminemia

            (4) Pulmonary atelectasis

            (5) Malignancy

            (6) Constrictive pericarditis

        b. Exudates

            (1) Pulmonary embolism

            (2) Bacterial pneumonia

            (3) Tuberculosis

          (4) Malignancies

              (a) Primary pleural

              (b) Metastatic

          (5) Dressler's syndrome

          (6) GI Disease

              (a) Esophageal perforation

              (b) Pancreatitis

          (7) Intra-abdominal abscess

3. Grossly bloody pleural effusions
   (RBCs >100,000/μL)

    a. Etiologies

        (1) Trauma

        (2) Pulmonary infarction

        (3) Malignancy

4. *Pleural Empyema*

    a. DEFINITION

        (1) A collection of pus within the pleural cavity with or without a broncho-pleural fistula.

        (2) Etiologies

            (a) Infections

                ▸ **50% are secondary to pneumonia**

                ▸ Abscess

                    • Lung abscess

                    • Subphrenic abscess

                ▸ Tuberculosis

                ▸ Fungal infections

            (b) Chest trauma, especially penetrating chest wounds

            (c) Spontaneous pneumothorax

B. DIAGNOSIS

    1. History and physical

        a. Weight loss

        b. Persistent or low-grade fever

        c. Night sweats

        d. Cough

        e. Chest pain

        f. Tachypnea

        g. Diminished or absent breath sounds over the effusion

    2. Laboratory

        a. Thoracentesis to obtain the pleural fluid and establish the diagnosis

            (1) Transudates

                (a) Clear fluid

(b) Protein <3.0 g/dL

(c) LDH <200 IU/L

(d) Glucose >60 mg/dL

(e) Leukocytes <1000 cells/mm³

(f) Specific gravity <1.016

(2) Exudates

(a) Clear, cloudy or bloody fluid

(b) Protein >3.0 g/dL

(c) LDH >200 IU/L

(d) Glucose <60 mg/dL

(e) Leukocytes >1000 cells/mm³

(f) Specific gravity >1.016

(3) Empyema

(a) WBC count >10,000 cells/mm³

(b) + Gram stain

(c) + cultures

(d) Glucose >40 mg/dL

(e) pH <7.2

b. Chest X-ray

AP and lateral decubitus for diagnosis and to monitor effusion

c. Biopsy

(1) Malignancy

(2) TB is suspected

3. TREATMENT

a. Transudates and exudates

Treat the underlying pathology

b. Empyema

(1) **The key to treatment is adequate drainage**.

(a) Drain it with a chest tube

(b) Inadequate drainage with a chest tube, then surgery may be required

(2) It will not respond to antibiotic therapy alone

III. CHRONIC OBSTRUCTIVE PULMONARY DISEASE

A. *Asthma*

1. DEFINITION

a. Asthma is a chronic disease characterized by airway *hyperresponsiveness*.

(1) Recurrent spasms of the muscles of the bronchi and bronchioles.

Symptoms of wheezing and breathlessness

(2) Edema of the lower airway structures

(3) A marked ↑ in bronchial mucous.

b. The result is mild to severe obstruction to airflow in the tracheobronchial tree.

c. **Status Asthmaticus is obstruction lasting for days or weeks.**

d. Viral infections and allergens are two of the major triggers in childhood asthma.

e. ↑ morbidity

Underdiagnosis and inappropriate treatment

f. Asthma can be divided into

(1) *Extrinsic Asthma*

(a) An IgE-mediated response.

▸ Airborne allergens

▸ Animal dander

▸ Foods

(2) *Intrinsic Asthma*

(a) Nonallergic (Non-IgE) etiology.

▸ Irritant exposure

• Pollution

• Fumes

• Tobacco smoke

▸ Infection

▸ Gastroesophageal reflux

(3) *Mixed Asthma*

A combination of both.

(4) *Occupational Asthma*

(a) Toluene di-isocyanate

(b) Platinum

(c) Nickel

(5) *Drug-induced*

(a) Aspirin

Many of these patients have nasal polyps

2. DIAGNOSIS

a. **"All that wheezes is not asthma"**

b. A good *history* is essential

(1) Wheezing

(2) Shortness of breath

(3) Dyspnea

(4) Cough

(5) ↑ sputum production

(6) Chest tightness

c. A good *physical* exam is essential

(1) Wheezing

(2) ↑ expiratory phase

(3) Tachypnea

(4) Cyanosis

       (5) Use of accessory respiratory muscles

       (6) Tachycardia

       (7) Pulsus paradoxus

   d. Laboratory

       (1) Pulmonary function studies reveal an "obstructive" pattern

       (2) ± eosinophilia on CBC

       (3) ± ↑ levels of IgE

       (4) Sputum exam

           Casts of small airway

       (5) Arterial blood gases

           Hypoxemia during an episode

       (6) Chest X-ray

          (1) ± hyperinflation

          (2) ± patchy infiltrates secondary to atelectasis.

3. TREATMENT

   a. **Avoidance of triggers**

   b. Beta-adrenergic agonists

       (1) Epinephrine

       (2) Albuterol

       (3) Terbutaline

       (4) Metaproterenol

       (5) Pirbuterol

   c. Theophyllines

   d. Anti-inflammatories

       (1) Corticosteroids

          (a) Inhaled

             ▸ Beclomethasone dipropionate

             ▸ Triamcinolone acetonide

             ▸ Flunisolide

          (b) Systemic

       (2) Cromolyn sodium

       (3) Nedocromil sodium

   e. Anticholinergics

       (1) Aerosolized atropine

       (2) Ipratropium bromide

B. *Chronic Bronchitis*

  1. DEFINITION

   a. Chronic bronchitis is characterized by a *chronic productive cough* for at least three months in a year, for two successive years.

   b. Cigarette smoking is the most important risk factor in development of chronic bronchitis and is commonly seen in smokers over the age of forty.

2. DIAGNOSIS "The Blue Bloater"
    a. **Chronic productive cough**
    b. Cyanosis
    c. Often obese
    d. Rhonchi and wheezes
    e. Intermittent dyspnea
    f. Pedal edema
    g. Chest X-ray
        ↑ bronchovascular markings and cardiomegaly
    h. Abnormal pulmonary function studies
        (1) ↓ maximal expiratory flow rates
        (2) ↑ residual volume
    i. Arterial blood gases
        (1) Hypercapnia
        (2) Hypoxemia
    j. **Episodes of respiratory failure are common**
3. TREATMENT
    a. **Stop Smoking**
    b. Beta-adrenergic agonists
    c. Anticholinergics
    d. Theophyllines
    e. Inhaled corticosteroids
    f. Antibiotics
        For acute exacerbations
    g. Mucolytics and expectorants
    h. Oxygen therapy (1-2 L/min.)
        (1) *Hypoxemia drives their respiration.*
            ↑ the pO_2 will ↓ respiratory rate and cause further ↑ CO_2 and eventually, they stop breathing.
    i. Prophylaxis
        (1) Influenza A and B vaccine
        (2) Pneumococcal vaccine
C. *Emphysema*
  1. DEFINITION
    a. Emphysema is characterized by destruction of the alveolar septa and distention of the air spaces *distal* to the terminal bronchioles.
    b. Cigarette smoking is the most important risk factor in development of emphysema.
    c. Etiologies
        (1) Panacinar
            Due to *Alpha-1-antitrysin deficiency*.

           (2) Centrilobular
               (a) **Cigarette smoking**
               (b) Pollution
               (c) Occupational
                    Firefighters

2. DIAGNOSIS "The Pink Puffer"
    a. Minimal cough and sputum
    b. ↑ exertional dyspnea
    c. Pursed lip breathing
    d. Use of accessory muscles to breathe
    e. Breath sounds diminished
    f. Barrel-shaped chest
    g. Asthenic body
    h. Prolonged expiratory phase of breathing
    i. Tachypnea
    j. Pulmonary function studies
            ↓ maximal flow rates
    k. Arterial blood gases
        Mild hypoxemia
    l. Chest X-ray
        (1) Small heart
        (2) Hyperinflation
        (3) Flat diaphragms
        (4) Bullous changes

3. TREATMENT
    a. **Stop Smoking**
    b. Beta-adrenergic agonists
        (1) Albuterol
        (2) Terbutaline
        (3) Metaproterenol
        (4) Pirbuterol
    c. Anticholinergics
    d. Theophyllines
    e. Inhaled corticosteroids
    f. Antibiotics
        For acute infections
    g. Mucolytics and expectorants
    h. Oxygen therapy (1-2 L/min.)
        (1) *Hypoxemia drives their respiration.*
            ↑ the pO_2 will ↓ respiratory rate and cause further ↑ CO_2 and eventually, they stop breathing.

          i. Prophylaxis
              (1) Influenza A and B vaccine
              (2) Pneumococcal vaccine

IV. LUNG CANCER
    A. Etiologies
        1. **Smoking (>90%)**
        2. Asbestos exposure
        3. Radiation
        4. Hydrocarbons
        5. Heavy metals
        6. Chronic interstitial pneumonitis
    B. Approximately 90% of lung cancers are "bronchogenic carcinomas".
        1. *Non-small cell*
            a. Squamous cell (epidermoid) carcinoma
                (1) About 30% of all bronchogenic carcinomas
                (2) Location
                    66% hilar, 33% periphery
                (3) Cavitation is frequent
            b. Adenocarcinoma (including bronchoalveolar)
                (1) About 25% of all bronchogenic carcinomas
                (2) Location
                    Usually peripheral and tend to spread *hematogenously* to the CNS
                (3) ± cavitation
                (4) Bronchoalveolar carcinomas have a pneumonia-like infiltrate
            c. Large cell carcinoma
                (1) About 10% of all bronchogenic carcinomas
                (2) Location
                    Usually a larger peripheral lesion
                (3) Tends to cavitate
         2. *Small cell*
            a. Small cell carcinoma (including "Oat cell")
                (1) About 20% of all bronchogenic carcinomas
                (2) Location
                    Usually hilar with early mediastinal involvement
                (3) No cavitation
        3. DIAGNOSIS
            a. 5-15% are detected when the patient is asymptomatic
            b. History and physical
                (1) **Cough**

(2) Weight loss

(3) Dyspnea

(4) Chest pain

(5) Hemoptysis

(6) 10-50% of bronchogenic carcinomas present with a paraneoplastic syndrome

c. Laboratory

(1) CXR/CT/MRI

To identify the location of lesion and identify mediastinal nodes.

(2) Tissue diagnosis by:

(a) Bronchoscopy with biopsy

(b) Needle biopsy under fluoroscopy or CT

(c) Mediastinoscopy

(d) Thoracotomy

4. TREATMENT

a. Non-small cell

(1) Resectable

(a) Surgery

(b) Radiation therapy

(c) Chemotherapy

b Nonresectable non-small cell and small cell

(1) Radiation therapy

(2) Chemotherapy

5. PROGNOSIS

5-year survival for all patients 8-12%.

V. **INTERSTITIAL LUNG DISEASE**

A. Pneumoconioses

1. DEFINITION

The *inhalation* of organic dust causing a chronic noninfectious inflammatory response of the alveolar wall that separates the capillary endothelial cells from the alveolar epithelial cells.

2. DIAGNOSIS

a. Inhaled substances

(1) Metals

(a) Iron

(b) Aluminum

(c) Beryllium

(2) Nonfibrous minerals

(a) **Coal**

▸ Black lung

- Simple coal-workers' pneumonconiosis
  - ↑ cough
  - Fine diffuse reticulonodular pattern on CXR.
  - Little functional impairment
- Complicated coal-workers' pneumonconiosis
  - ↑ fibrosis
  - Restrictive lung disease
  - Nodular densities on chest X-ray

(b) Silica

(2) Fibrous minerals

    (a) Talc

    (b) Fiber glass

    (c) **Asbestos**

- ▸ History and physical
  - Insidious onset of dyspnea
  - Chronic nonproductive cough
  - A history of exposure at least a decade earlier
  - Chest pain
  - Clubbing
- ▸ Laboratory
  - Biopsy
    - Diffuse interstitial focal, mucosal, and bronchiolar fibrosis.
    - "Asbestos bodies"
    - Pleural thickening and calcification
  - Arterial blood gases
    - Hypoxemia
- ▸ Pulmonary Function studies
  - Restrictive disease characterized by
    - ↓ vital, total lung and diffusing capacity
- ▸ Chest X-ray
  - Early
    - Ground-glass appearance, ± fine stippling
  - Later
    - Basilar fibrosis, pleural thickening, calcific pleural plaques, bilateral pleural effusion.

3. TREATMENT
   - a. Stop smoking
   - b. Supplemental oxygen
   - c. Bronchodilators, if indicated
   - d. Aggressive management of infections

4. PROGNOSIS
    a. Asbestosis
        (1) Severity = length of exposure
        (2) ↑ risk tuberculosis in smokers
        (3) ↑ risk of lung cancer in smokers
        (4) ↑ risk of mesothelioma
        (5) **This illness is chronic, progressive and irreversible.**

B. *Sarcoidosis*
   1. DEFINITION
      Sarcoidosis is a multisystem *granulomatous* disease of unknown etiology.
   2. DIAGNOSIS
      a. History and physical
          (1) Fatigue
          (2) Weight loss
          (3) Cough
          (4) Dyspnea
          (5) Lymphadenopathy
          (6) Night sweats
          (7) Facial rash
          (8) ± erythema nodosum.
          (9) **The patient may also be asymptomatic.**
      b. Laboratory
          (1) ↑ alkaline phosphatase
          (2) 50% have a leukopenia with lymphopenia or anemia
          (3) ↑ angiotensin-converting enzyme
          (4) Hypercalcemia and hypercalciuria
          (5) Hypergammaglobulinemia seen primarily in black patients
          (6) 50% have an abnormal ECG
          (7) **Chest X-ray**
             (a) Perihilar and peritracheal lymph nodes
             (b) Interstitial infiltrates
             (c) Interstitial fibrosis.
             (d) Bronchoscopy or mediastinoscopy with biopsy
                ▸ **Noncaseating epithelioid granulomas.**
   3. TREATMENT
      a. Asymptomatic
         No treatment is necessary
      b. Symptomatic
          (1) **Systemic corticosteroids**
          (2) Chloroquine
          (3) Azathioprine

    (4) Indomethacin

    (5) Methotrexate

  4. PROGNOSIS

    (1) 33% make a total recovery

    (2) 33% recover with minimal changes

    (3) 25% have significant morbidity and disability

    (4) 10% die with their illness

    (5) Generally, ↑ number of systems involved, the worse the prognosis

VI. PULMONARY EMBOLUS

  A. DEFINITION

    1. Pulmonary Embolism is an event in which a deep vein thrombus of the lower extremity dislodges and enters the pulmonary circulation.

    2. **All of the etiologies reflect a hypercoagulable state.**

      a. Primary (Inherited)

        (1) Antithrombin III deficiency

        (2) Protein S deficiency

        (3) Protein C deficiency

        (4) Excessive plasminogen activator inhibitor.

        (5) Dysfibrinogenemia

      b. Secondary (Acquired)

        (1) Trauma

        (2) Immobilization

        (3) Surgery

        (4) Cancer

        (5) Oral contraceptives

        (6) Pregnancy

        (7) Obesity

        (8) Congestive heart failure

        (9) MI

        (10) Sepsis

        (11) Stroke

        (12) Polycythemia

  B. DIAGNOSIS

    1. History and physical

      a. **Dyspnea**

      b. Tachypnea

      c. Anxiety

      d. Tachycardia

      e. Chest pain

      f. Accentuated P_2

g. Low grade temperature

h. Syncope (in severe cases)

i. Hypotension (in severe cases)

2. Laboratory

a. **Arterial blood gases are unreliable as a screening test.**

b. Electrocardiogram

(1) Rule out MI

(2) Check for right heart strain

c. **Chest X-ray may be normal. It does not rule out PE.**

d. **V/Q (Ventilation/perfusion) lung scan is the procedure of choice for diagnosis.**

e. ± scans can be followed by pulmonary arteriography if necessary for diagnosis.

f. Evaluation for deep vein thrombosis

(1) **Venography**

(2) Doppler ultrasonography

(3) Venous duplex scanning

(4) Impedance plethysmography

C. TREATMENT

1. Anticoagulation

a. Heparin therapy, stat.

b. Coumadin therapy to begin 12-24 hours after beginning heparin therapy.

c. **Contraindications**

(1) Bleeding diathesis

(2) Stroke (hemorrhagic)

(3) Trauma

(4) Surgery/postpartum

2. Systemic thrombolytic therapy

a. Medications

(1) Urokinase

(2) Streptokinase

(3) Recombinant tissue plasminogen activator

b. ± reduction in mortality

3. Inferior Vena Cava filters

4. Pulmonary embolectomy

VII. **SLEEP APNEA**

A. DEFINITION

1. Repetitive episodes of *apnea* (cessation of airflow >10 seconds) during sleep.

2. Etiologies

a. Central

(1) Loss of neural drive during sleep

(2) Rare

b. Obstructive
- (1) Upper airway obstruction
- (2) Common

c. Underlying medical disorders
- (1) COPD
- (2) Hypertension
- (3) Hypothyroidism

B. DIAGNOSIS
1. History and physical
    a. **Excessive daytime sleepiness**
    b. **Snoring**
    c. Waking up gasping for air
    d. Observed apneas at night
    e. Fatigue
    f. Forgetfulness
    g. Obesity
    h. Nasal or oropharyngeal tissue enlargement causing obstruction
2. Laboratory
    a. Sleep study (polysomnogram)
    - (1) Multiple episodes of apnea
    - (2) Oxygen desaturation and hypoxemia
    - (3) There may be observed cardiac arrhythmias
    b. Evaluation for predisposing conditions

C. TREATMENT
1. Correction of exacerbating factors
    a. Correction of obesity
    b. Avoidance of sedatives and alcohol
    c. Appropriate treatment of underlying medical disorders
2. **Nasal CPAP**
3. Protriptyline at bedtime for central and mixed apneas
4. Surgery
    a. Surgery to remove excessive or hypertrophied tissues causing obstruction
    b. Tracheostomy (for very severe disease)

I. CORONARY HEART DISEASE
A. DEFINITION
1. *Atherosclerotic heart disease*

The formation of atheromata in the small and medium arteries of the heart leading to ↓ blood flow and ↑ myocardial ischemia.

2. **Angina pectoris is the clinical expression (syndrome) brought about by the ↑ myocardial ischemia.**

   a. Ischemia occurs when the demand for oxygen by the myocardial tissues exceeds the supply.

   b. *Classic angina*

   A substernal ache, heaviness or pressure precipitated by activity or emotional upset

   c. *Variant (Prinzmetal) angina*

   (1) A substernal ache, heaviness or pressure not related to exercise or stress.

   (2) It occurs at rest, after exercise or at night during sleep.

   d. *Unstable (Crescendo or Preinfarction) angina*

   (1) Anginal pain which has changed in character, duration or frequency

   (2) The pain is severe, prolonged, and precipitated by little or no exercise and may occur during sleep.

   (3) It is usually *unresponsive* to a single nitroglycerin tablet.

   e. *Silent ischemia*

   Patients with evidence of CAD diagnosed by ECG or stress tests *should be treated* even if they are not having signs and symptoms of angina.

3. Risk factors: "HEART'S LOAD"

   a. H = Hypertension (Essential or secondary)

   b. E = ECG abnormalities

   c. A = Activity (sedentary life style)

   d. R = Relatives (family history)

   e. T = Type A personality

   f. S = Smoking

   g. L = Lipids

   h. O = Obesity

   i. A = Age (↑ atherosclerosis with age)

   j. D = Diabetes mellitus (small vessel disease)

B. DIAGNOSIS
1. History and physical

   a. A substernal ache, squeezing, heaviness or pressure precipitated by activity or emotional upset.

   b. Radiation of the pain to left arm, neck, jaw or abdomen

   c. Diaphoresis

   d. Nausea

e. Anxiety
2. Laboratory
   a. **The resting ECG may or not be diagnostic.**
   b. Many times there are only nonspecific S-T wave changes and not the classic *S-T wave depression* during an episode.
   c. The resting ECG in variant angina reveals S-T wave elevation during an episode.
   d. Exercise "stress" ECG
   e. Stress echocardiography
   f. Stress thallium scan
   g. Coronary angiography

C. TREATMENT
   1. Nitrates
      a. Reduce coronary artery resistance
      b. Dilate the peripheral vessels
   2. Beta-blockers
      a. Useful in patients with exercise induced angina by keeping pulse approximately 60 beats/minute.
      b. Good in controlling palpitations, sinus tachycardia and diaphoresis.
      c. ↓ Sudden cardiac death *after* MI
      d. **Don't use beta-blockers in bronchospastic disease.**
   3. Calcium channel blockers
      a. Benefit for both stable and unstable angina
      b. Vasodilate the coronary and peripheral circulation
      c. They prevent coronary artery spasm
   4. Treatment of underlying medical conditions
   5. ↓ risk factors
   6. Low fat diet
   7. Heparin therapy
      Unstable angina only
   8. Surgery
      a. Percutaneous transluminal coronary angioplasty (balloon angioplasty)
      b. Coronary bypass surgery

II. **HYPERTENSION**
   A. DEFINITION
      1. A sustained elevation of the systolic pressure of >140 mm Hg and/or
      2. A sustained elevation of the diastolic pressure of >90 mm Hg.
      3. >90% of hypertension is primary or "essential"
      4. Malignant hypertension
         a. Diastolic pressure >130 mm Hg.

      b. Retinopathy ± papilledema

      c. Necrosis of arterioles and small arteries.

5. Systolic hypertension is a sustained elevation of systolic pressure >160 mm Hg.

6. Secondary hypertension

      a. Renal

            (1) Renal artery stenosis

            (2) Acute and chronic glomerulonephritis

            (3) Chronic pyelonephritis

            (4) Polycystic kidney disease

      b. Endocrine

            (1) Diseases of the adrenal cortex and medulla.

                  (a) Primary hyperaldosteronism

                        Mineralocorticoid excess

                  (b) Cushing's disease

                        Glucocorticoid excess

                  (c) Adrenogenital syndromes

                        Enzyme defects

                  (d) Pheochromocytoma

                        Catecholamines

            (2) Diseases of the thyroid gland

                  (a) Hyperthyroidism

                  (b) Myxedema

            (3) Diseases of the pituitary

                Acromegaly

            (4) Diseases of the pancreas

                Diabetes mellitus

      c. Vascular

          Coarctation of the aorta

      d. Neurologic

            (1) Acute ↑ intracranial pressure

            (2) Spinal cord transection

      e. Drug-induced

            (1) Sympathomimetics

            (2) Oral contraceptives

            (3) Corticosteroids

            (4) Decongestants

      f. Miscellaneous

         Pregnancy

B. DIAGNOSIS

    1. A *good history* is essential

        a. Coronary risk factors

        b. Family history

   2. A *complete physical examination* is essential

        a. Fundoscopic examination

        b. Three ↑ BP readings on different occasions

        c. Auscultation of the heart for murmurs and extra sounds

        d. Pulses and bruits

   3. Laboratory

        a. CBC

        b. Chemistry-28

             (1) The most cost effective way of obtaining

                (a) Potassium

                (b) Calcium

                (c) Glucose

                (d) Cholesterol

                (e) Creatinine

                (f) Uric acid

        c. Urinalysis

        d. Some also advocate

             (1) ECG

             (2) Chest X-ray

        e. Special testing for secondary hypertension only if there is a ↑ index of suspicion from history, physical, or laboratory.

C. TREATMENT

   1. Nonpharmacologic

        a. Weight reduction

        b. Smoking cessation

        c. ↑ exercise

        d. ↓ sodium

        e. ↓ alcohol

        f. ↓ fats in diet

        g. ↓ stress

   2. Pharmacologic

        a. Diuretics

        b. ACE inhibitors

        c. Calcium channel blockers

        d. Beta-blockers

        e. Vasodilators

        f. Centrally acting adrenergic inhibitors

D. COMPLICATIONS
  1. Central nervous system
      a. Cerebrovascular accident
      b. Subarachnoid hemorrhage
  2. Renal disease
      Chronic renal failure
  3. Heart and vessels
      a. Coronary artery disease
      b. Congestive heart failure
      c. Aortic aneurysm

III. ACUTE MYOCARDIAL INFARCTION
  A. DEFINITION
      Occlusion of a coronary vessel by a thrombus with resulting *irreversible* myocardial necrosis.
  B. DIAGNOSIS
  1. History
      a. **Crushing substernal chest pain**
          (1) The pain can radiate to the left arm, neck, jaw, back and abdomen.
          (2) The pain is *not relieved* with rest or nitroglycerin.
          (3) **About a quarter of acute MIs are silent.**
      b. Dyspnea
      c. Anxiety
      d. Nausea and vomiting
      e. Syncope
  2. Physical
      a. Diaphoresis
      b. Weakness
      c. Pallor
      d. Cough
      e. Wheezes, crackles
      f. Tachycardia or bradycardia
      g. S_4 gallop
      h. Jugular venous distention
      i. ↓ BP
      j. Irregular pulse
  3. Laboratory
      a. ECG
          (1) *Q wave MI*
              Acute elevation of ST wave which evolves into T-wave depression and the formation of Q-waves hours later.

(2) *Non-Q-wave MI*

Acute ST wave depression which evolves into persistent changes (major or minor) of the ST or T-wave *without* the formation of Q-waves.

(3) **Even in the face of a negative ECG, if there is a high index of suspicion hospitalize the patient for monitoring and evaluation.**

(4) Serial ECGs for three days

b. Enzyme studies (x3 days)

(1) CPK isoenzymes

↑ of CK-MB isoenzyme peaks at ≈24 hrs

(2) ↑ of SGOT peaks at ≈18 to 36 hours

(3) ↑ of LDH peaks at ≈3 to 6 days

c. ↑ WBC

d. ↑ sedimentation rate

4. Mortality is greatest within the first two hours of signs and symptoms

5. **There will be signs of cardiogenic shock if > 40% of the myocardium is infarcted.**

C. TREATMENT

1. Hospitalize
2. IV line
3. Analgesia
4. Oxygen
5. Sedation
6. Soft diet
7. Beta-blockers
8. Anticoagulation
9. Thrombolytic therapy
   a. Streptokinase
   b. tPA (Tissue plasminogen activator)
10. Angioplasty
11. Supervised cardiac rehabilitation

D. COMPLICATIONS

1. Cardiogenic shock
2. Congestive heart failure
3. Dysrhythmia
4. Ventricular aneurysm
5. Dressler's syndrome
6. Pericarditis

IV. CONGESTIVE HEART FAILURE
  A. DEFINITION
1. A condition by which the heart is unable to deliver the requisite amount of blood to meet the metabolic demands of the body either at activity or rest.
2. Etiologies
    a. Coronary artery disease
    b. Hypertension
    c. Myocardial infarction
    d. Valvular disease
    e. Cardiomyopathies
  B. DIAGNOSIS
1. History
    a. **The most common triad of complaints are respiratory**.
      (1) Dyspnea
      (2) Orthopnea
      (3) Paroxysmal nocturnal dyspnea
    b. Fatigue
    c. Tachypnea
2. Physical
    a. Peripheral edema
    b. Crackles and wheezes (Cardiac asthma)
    c. Pleural effusion
    d. Pulmonary congestion/edema
    e. Hepatomegaly
    f. S_3 gallop
    g. Jugular venous distention
    h. Cardiomegaly
    i. Tachycardia
3. Laboratory
    a. Baseline
      (1) CBC
      (2) Chem-28
      (3) Urinalysis
    b. ECG
      No specific findings in CHF. Underlying disease may be identified.
    c. Chest X-ray
      (1) Early Changes
        (a) ↑ heart size
        (b) ↑ blood flow to upper lobes

(2) Mid- to late changes

     (a) Interstitial edema

     (b) Kerley's B lines

     (c) Pleural effusion

     (d) Classic "butterfly" pattern of pulmonary edema.

  d. Echocardiography

    Valuable in diagnosing *underlying cardiac disease* leading to CHF.

C. TREATMENT

1. Nonpharmacologic

  a. Moderate activity

  b. Diet

    (1) Salt restriction

    (2) Weight loss

  c. Emotional support

2. Pharmacologic

  a. ↓ cardiac workload

    (1) Vasodilators

      ↓ the afterload

  b. ↓ excess fluid load

    (1) Diuretics

      ↓ the preload

  c. ↑ myocardial contraction

    Digoxin/digitalis

  d. ACE inhibitors

  e. ± lidocaine for tachyarrythmias

  f. Sympathomimetic amines (severe CHF)

    (1) Dopamine

    (2) Dobutamine

    (3) Amrinone

  g. Surgical correction of underlying cardiac lesion

  h. Transplantation

V. ARRHYTHMIAS

A. ATRIAL ARRHYTHMIAS

1. *Sinus Bradycardia*

  a. DEFINITION

    (1) A heart rate < 60 beats/minute.

    (2) Etiology

      (a) It may be physiologic (athletes)

      (b) ↑ intracranial pressure

(c) Coronary artery disease

(d) Hypothyroidism

b. DIAGNOSIS

(1) May be asymptomatic

(2) Lightheadedness and dizziness

(3) Syncope

(4) ECG

(a) P waves are normal

(b) PR interval normal or prolonged

(c) QRS is normal

c. TREATMENT

(1) None if mild

(2) Treatment of underlying disease process

(3) Severe disease

(a) Atropine

(b) Pacemaker

2. *Sinus Tachycardia*

a. DEFINITION

(1) A heart rate >100 beats/minute

(2) Typically not >170 beats/minute

(3) Etiology

(a) Infection

(b) Hypovolemia

(c) Anxiety/pain

(d) Hypoxemia

(e) Hyperthyroidism

(f) ↑ catecholamines

b. DIAGNOSIS

(1) ECG

(a) P waves are normal

(b) PR interval normal or slightly shortened

(c) QRS is normal

c. TREATMENT

Treatment of underlying disease process

3. *Paroxysmal Supraventricular Tachycardia*

a. DEFINITION

PSVT arises from a sustained reentry mechanism involving the SA node, the atrium and the AV node.

b. DIAGNOSIS
- (1) Begins suddenly with ↑ heart rate
  - (a) ↑ anxiety
  - (b) ± palpitations
  - (c) Shortness of breath
  - (d) Weakness and/or dizziness
  - (e) ± chest pain.
- (2) Atrial rate = 140-250 contractions/minute
- (3) **AV nodal reentry tachycardia is the most common form of PSVT**
  - (a) Typical
    - ▸ P waves are hidden in the QRS complex
    - ▸ Atrial and ventricular ratio 1:1
    - ▸ Abrupt onset and termination
    - ▸ Most patients *do not* have underlying cardiac disease.
  - (b) Atypical
    - ▸ P waves are inverted in the T wave
    - ▸ P wave is normal or slightly prolonged
    - ▸ Abrupt onset and termination

c. TREATMENT
- (1) Vagal maneuvers
- (2) IV adenosine
- (3) IV verapamil
- (4) Beta-blockers
- (5) Cardioversion if unresponsive

4. *Premature Atrial Contractions*

a. DEFINITION
- (1) Ectopic foci in the atria generate multiple, usually premature impulses.
- (2) Etiology
  - (a) Drug induced
    - ▸ Alcohol
    - ▸ Nicotine
    - ▸ Stimulants
  - (b) Fatigue
  - (c) Anxiety
  - (d) CHF
  - (e) Electrolyte imbalance
  - (f) Hypoxia
  - (g) Infection

b. DIAGNOSIS

(1) May be asymptomatic

(2) Feeling of "missed" or skipped beats

(3) ECG

A benign rhythm characterized by *abnormal P-waves* and a *compensatory pause* after the atrial premature beat.

c. TREATMENT

(1) Treatment of underlying disease process

(2) ± beta-blockers

(3) ± calcium channel blockers

5. *Multifocal Atrial Tachycardia*

a. DEFINITION

Multifocal impulses arise in the atria, irregularly at an ↑ rate

b. DIAGNOSIS

(1) Atrial rate = 130-200 beats/minute

(2) ECG

>3 *different* P waves with varying PR intervals

(3) Associated with advanced pulmonary disease.

c. TREATMENT

(1) Correct the underlying hypoxia

(2) Verapamil to slow ventricular rate

6. *Atrial Flutter*

a. DEFINITION

(1) An ectopic atrial foci releases impulses at a rate of 250-350 contractions per minute.

(2) The rate is so fast the AV node is only capable of transmitting the impulse to the ventricles at a 2:1, 3:1 or 4:1 ratio, hence, a 2:1, 3:1, or 4:1 block.

(3) Etiology

(a) Usually as the result of organic heart disease.

▸ Mitral stenosis

▸ Atrial septal defect

▸ Coronary artery disease

(b) Hypertension

(c) Hyperthyroidism

(d) COPD

b. DIAGNOSIS

(1) ECG

(a) **P waves are identical producing a *saw-tooth* pattern.**

(b) The QRS is normal.

c. TREATMENT

    (1) Treatment of underlying disease process

    (2) Control of atrial rate

        (a) DC cardioversion in the presence of clinical instability

        (b) Quinidine, procainamide, disopyramide to convert to sinus rhythm

        (c) Atrial overdrive pacing

    (3) ↓ ventricular rate

        (a) Digoxin

        (b) Beta-blocker

        (c) Verapamil

    (4) ± anticoagulation

    (5) If medication fails, DC cardioversion.

7. *Atrial Fibrillation*

  a. DEFINITION

    (1) Multiple atrial foci release impulses at a rate of >300 contractions per minute. The ventricular response is irregularly irregular at a rate of 120-160 beats/minute

    (2) Etiology

        (a) Usually as the result of organic heart disease

            ‣ Mitral stenosis

            ‣ Atrial septal defect

            ‣ Coronary artery disease

        (b) Hypertension

        (c) Hyperthyroidism

        (d) COPD

        (e) Hypoxia

        (f) Pulmonary embolism

        (g) Pericarditis

  b. DIAGNOSIS

    (1) Signs and symptoms

        (a) Palpitations

        (b) Rapid irregular pulse

        (c) Dizziness

        (d) Dyspnea

        (e) Syncope

    (2) ECG

        (a) P-Waves are not identified

        (b) Usually normal, irregularly spaced QRS complex

    c. TREATMENT
        (1) Atrial fibrillation + rapid ventricular response + worsening clinical picture
            (hypotension, ischemia, heart failure, MI) → DC cardioversion
        (2) ↓ ventricular rate
            (a) Digoxin
            (b) Beta-blocker
            (c) Calcium channel blockers
        (3) Conversion to sinus rhythm
            (a) Chemical cardioversion
                Quinidine or procainamide
            (b) DC cardioversion
        (4) **Anticoagulation to ↓ risk of stroke**
        (5) Failure of drug therapy, DC cardioversion.
B. VENTRICULAR ARRHYTHMIAS
    1. *Ventricular Premature Contractions*
        a. DEFINITION
            (1) One or more ectopic foci located in the ventricle produce impulses which
                cause an out of sequence contraction.
            (2) Etiologies
                (a) It may occur in normal individuals
                    ‣ Fatigue
                    ‣ Anxiety
                    ‣ Alcohol and/or caffeine
                (b) Hypoxia
                (c) Myocardial infarction
                    The ↑ size of the infarct, the ↑ frequency of the VPCs
                (d) Ischemia
                (e) CHF
                (f) Hypokalemia
                (g) Drugs
                    ‣ Digitalis toxicity
                    ‣ Tricyclics
                    ‣ Phenothiazines
                    ‣ Quinidine
        b. DIAGNOSIS
            (1) ECG
                (a) Wide bizarre QRS complex
                (b) T wave is oriented in the opposite direction to its QRS complex
                (c) Bigeminy.......... every other beat is a VPC.
                (d) Trigeminy........ every third beat is a VPC.

(e) Couplet or pair......... two successive VPCs.
   (2) VPCs are worrisome if
      (a) Multifocal
      (b) "R on T phenomenon"
          R wave on the VPC falls on the T wave of the preceding beat.
      (c) Runs of VPCs
      (d) >6 per minute
  c. TREATMENT
    (1) Treat the underlying illness or discontinue the medication
    (2) Only very symptomatic patients need to be treated
    (3) Beta-blockers
    (4) IV lidocaine or procainamide for VPCs after MI
2. *Ventricular Tachycardia*
  a. DEFINITION
    (1) >3 or more *successive* VPCs at a rate of between 100-250 beats/minute
    (2) The most commonly encountered *life-threatening* arrhythmia
    (3) Etiologies
      (a) Acute MI
      (b) CHF
      (c) Ischemia
      (d) Digitalis toxicity
  b. DIAGNOSIS
    (1) ECG
      (a) Wide bizarre QRS complex
      (b) T wave is oriented in the opposite direction to its QRS complex
    (2) Unsustained VT
      Terminates spontaneously in <30 seconds
    (3) Sustained VT
      >30 seconds or causes hemodynamic collapse.
    (4) A tachycardia with a wide QRS, think VT if
      (a) Fusion complexes
      (b) AV dissociation
      (c) Left axis deviation
    (5) Torsades de Pointes
      (a) VT at a rate of 200-250 beats/minute where the complexes seem to rotate around an imaginary point or isoelectric line.
         It may occur following quinidine, procainamide or disopyramide administration.

(b) Treatment
- ‣ Clinically unstable
  - • DC cardioversion
- ‣ Discontinue the medication stat
- ‣ Magnesium sulfate
- ‣ Temporary pacing

c. TREATMENT

(1) DC cardioversion if unstable

(2) IV lidocaine and/or procainamide and/or bretylium

(3) Second line drugs, mexiletine and amiodarone may be needed.

(4) If drug therapy is unsuccessful, implantable defibrillator or surgery.

(5) Prognosis for sustained VT is poor

3. *Ventricular Fibrillation*

a. DEFINITION

(1) QRS and T waves are replaced by variable low-amplitude wave forms

(2) The heart quivers and there is no effective emptying of the ventricles.

(3) Etiologies

(a) MI

(b) AV block

(c) Ischemia

b. DIAGNOSIS

Irregular oscillations without the presence of P waves, QRS complexes, or T waves.

c. TREATMENT

(1) Immediate DC cardioversion

(2) IV Lidocaine

(3) Correction of physiologic abnormalities secondary to VF.

(4) Chronic therapy

(a) Amiodarone

(b) Implantation of automatic defibrillator

(5) Primary VF *within 72 hours* of acute MI is not associated with ↑ risk of recurrence.

C. CONDUCTION DISTURBANCES

1. AV block

a. *First-Degree Block*

(1) DEFINITION

A slowing or interruption of conduction between the atria and ventricles

(2) DIAGNOSIS

    (a) ECG

        Prolonged PR > 0.20 seconds

(3) TREATMENT

    None, may be normal variant or secondary to digitalis.

b. *Second-Degree Block*

    (1) Mobitz Type I

        (a) DEFINITION

- Narrow QRS + progressive ↑ of PR interval until a beat is dropped.
- Seen with digitalis toxicity and may occur with inferior MI.

        (b) TREATMENT

- None unless symptomatic, usually transient
- If symptomatic
  - Atropine
  - Temporary or permanent pacing

    (2) Mobitz Type II

        (a) DEFINITION

- A dangerous rhythm in which there is a block within or just below the bundle of His.

        (b) DIAGNOSIS

- ECG

    Wide QRS + fixed PR interval except with dropped beats

- Can be seen after acute anterior MI or with organic heart disease
- Can progress to complete heart block

        (c) TREATMENT

- Pacemaker

c. *Third-Degree Block*

    (1) DEFINITION

    The atria and the ventricles beat independently. There is no electrical activity transmitted through the AV node.

    (2) DIAGNOSIS

        (a) Most commonly seen after acute MI

        (b) Ominous if it occurs after anterior MI (indicative of large infarction)

        (c) Transient if it occurs after inferior-posterior MI

        (d) Can be seen with digitalis toxicity, ↑ levels of beta blockers and calcium channel blockers.

(e) ECG
- ► PR intervals vary
- ► P-P and R-R intervals are regular

(3) TREATMENT

Pacemaker, if not drug toxic or inferior-posterior infarction

2. *Wolff-Parkinson-White Syndrome*

a. DEFINITION

A *preexcitation syndrome* in which electrical activity from the atria is transmitted via an *alternate pathway* to the ventricles.

b. DIAGNOSIS

(1) Think supraventricular tachycardia + a delta wave

A delta wave is a slurred upstroke of QRS

(2) ECG

(a) A shortened PR interval of <.12 seconds

(b) A wide QRS complex

(c) A delta wave

(3) Can run the gamut from no symptoms to palpitations to syncope.

(4) Sudden death can occur.

c. TREATMENT

(1) Antiarrhythmics

(2) Cardioversion

(3) Pacemaker

(4) Surgical ablation

VI. VALVULAR HEART DISEASE

A. *Aortic Stenosis*

1. ETIOLOGY

a. **Congenital**

(1) The most common *congenital* lesion involving the outflow tract of the left ventricle.

(2) The valve is bicuspid.

b. Rheumatic

Always associated with mitral valve disease

c. Degenerative

2. DIAGNOSIS

a. Signs and symptoms

(1) 50% of patients with aortic stenosis have significant coronary artery disease

(2) Symptoms occur late

(a) Angina

(b) Syncope

(c) Left ventricular failure

(d) **The hallmark of aortic stenosis is the prominent crescendo-decrescendo murmur at the right sternal border.**

(e) S_4 common

(f) Pulsus parvus et tardus

A slowly rising carotid pulse which is sustained

(g) Carotid thrill

b. Laboratory

(1) ECG

(a) Left ventricular hypertrophy associated with S-T, T wave changes

(b) LBBB and Intraventricular conduction defects

(2) Chest X-ray

(a) Left ventricular enlargement

(b) Poststenotic dilation of the aorta

(c) Calcification of the valve

(3) Echocardiography

(a) Calcification and ↑ thickness of the valve

(b) Left ventricular hypertrophy

(4) Cardiac catheterization and angiography

(a) Document any regurgitation

(b) Evaluate the coronary arteries

(c) Calculate the effective aortic valve orifice size

3. TREATMENT

a. Antibiotic prophylaxis

b. Moderate physical activity

c. Treat the left ventricular failure

These patients depend on adequate preload, that is, ventricular filling, to drive their cardiac output.

d. Surgery

(1) Valvuloplasty

(2) Aortic valve replacement

B. *Aortic Regurgitation*

1. *Chronic Aortic Regurgitation*

a. ETIOLOGIES

(1) Infectious

(a) Rheumatic fever

(b) Syphilis

(c) Acute bacterial endocarditis

(2) Congenital

(3) Connective tissue diseases

(4) Hypertension
b. Chronic aortic insufficiency is well tolerated.
c. DIAGNOSIS
(1) Signs and symptoms
(a) Asymptomatic >4 decades because the left ventricle can compensate
(b) **Think symptoms of left ventricular failure**
- Exertional dyspnea
- Orthopnea
- Paroxysmal nocturnal dyspnea
(c) S_1 normal S_2 diminished
(d) **Blowing decrescendo diastolic murmur along the left sternal border.**
(e) Austin Flint murmur
A middiastolic or presystolic rumble best heard at the apex.
(f) Bounding pulses
(g) Widened pulse pressure
(h) S_3 common
(2) Laboratory
(a) ECG
Left ventricular hypertrophy
(b) Chest X-ray
- Left ventricular hypertrophy
- Prominent ascending aorta
(c) Echocardiogram
- Dilated, hyperdynamic left ventricle
- Left atrial enlargement
d. TREATMENT
(1) Treat the left ventricular failure
(2) Surgery
Valve replacement *before* irreversible left ventricular dilatation.
2. *Acute Aortic Insufficiency*
a. ETIOLOGIES
(1) Infective endocarditis
(2) Prosthetic valve malfunction
(3) Dissection of aorta
(4) Trauma
b. Acute aortic insufficiency is poorly tolerated.
c. DIAGNOSIS
(1) Signs and symptoms
(a) **Think left ventricular decompensation**

Dyspnea → pulmonary edema
- (b) Sinus tachycardia
- (c) Soft S_1 and S_2
- (d) Loud S_3 and absent S_4
- (e) **Low-pitched decrescendo diastolic murmur**
- (f) Austin Flint murmur
  - A middiastolic or presystolic rumble best heard at the apex.
- (g) Bibasilar crackles

(2) Laboratory
- (a) ECG
  - ‣ Sinus tachycardia
  - ‣ Left ventricular strain
- (b) Chest X-ray
  - Pulmonary edema with normal heart size.

(3) Echocardiography
- (a) Valvular abnormalities
- (b) Aortic root abnormalities can be identified.
- (c) Left ventricular end-diastolic volume not ↑ and left ventricular end-systolic volume is normal + a hyperdynamic contraction of the ventricle.

d. TREATMENT
- (1) **This is a life-threatening condition**
- (2) Treat the heart failure
- (3) Treat infection if it is present
- (4) Valvular surgery following preload and afterload reduction.

C. *Mitral Stenosis*

1. ETIOLOGIES
   - a. Rheumatic fever
   - b. Myxoma
   - c. Congenital

2. DIAGNOSIS
   - a. Signs and symptoms
     - (1) Asymptomatic until the third to fourth decade.
     - (2) Initial
       - (a) Fatigue
       - (b) ↑ exertional dyspnea
       - (c) Hemoptysis
       - (d) Cough
       - (e) Crackles
       - (f) Palpitations

(g) Initial loud S_1 which ↓ as stenosis ↑.

(h) Opening snap after S_2 ↓ as stenosis ↑.

(i) **Diastolic murmur in left lateral decubitus position**.

    (3) Later

        (a) Right ventricular enlargement, then failure

            ▸ Peripheral edema

            ▸ Hepatomegaly

            ▸ ↑ jugular distention

  b. Laboratory

    (1) ECG

        (a) Left atrial enlargement

        (b) Broad notched P waves

        (c) Atrial Fibrillation is common

        (d) Right ventricular hypertrophy

    (2) Chest X-ray

        (a) Left atrial enlargement

        (b) Right ventricular enlargement (late)

        (c) Valvular calcification (late)

        (d) Interstitial pulmonary edema (late)

    (3) Echocardiography

        (a) Thickening and calcification of the valve

        (b) Left atrial enlargement

3. TREATMENT

  a. Antibiotic prophylaxis

  b. Convert the atrial fibrillation if present

  c. Anticoagulation

  d. Treat the heart failure

  e. Surgery

    (1) Mitral percutaneous balloon valvuloplasty

    (2) Mitral valve replacement

D. *Mitral Regurgitation*

  1. *Chronic Mitral Regurgitation*

    a. ETIOLOGIES

      (1) Rheumatic fever

      (2) Coronary artery disease

      (3) Mitral valve prolapse

      (4) Infective endocarditis

      (5) Malfunction of prosthetic valve

      (6) Myxomatous degeneration

  b. DIAGNOSIS
    (1) Signs and symptoms
        (a) May be asymptomatic for decades
        (b) Left ventricular enlargement and then failure
        (c) Fatigue
        (d) Dyspnea
        (e) Crackles
        (f) Orthopnea
        (g) Dyspnea on exertion
        (h) **Holosystolic murmur, harsh, at the apex and radiating to the back or axilla**
        (i) Soft S_1
        (j) Widely split S_2
        (k) S_3 if there is severe regurgitation
    (2) Laboratory
        (a) ECG
            ‣ Left atrial enlargement
            ‣ Left ventricular hypertrophy
            ‣ Atrial fibrillation commonly
        (b) Chest X-ray
            ‣ Left atrial enlargement
            ‣ Left ventricular enlargement
            ‣ Interstitial edema
        (c) Echocardiogram
            ‣ Hyperdynamic dilated left ventricle
            ‣ Enlarged left atrium
            ‣ Valvular abnormalities
 c. TREATMENT
    (1) Antibiotic prophylaxis
    (2) Convert the atrial fibrillation if present.
    (3) Anticoagulation
    (4) Treat the heart failure
    (5) Surgery
        (a) Mitral valve reconstruction
        (b) Mitral valve replacement
2. *Acute Mitral Regurgitation*
 a. ETIOLOGIES
    (1) Ruptured chordae or papillary muscle
    (2) Leaflet perforation
    (3) Infective endocarditis

(4) Malfunction of prosthetic valve
b. DIAGNOSIS
    (1) Signs and symptoms
        (a) Acute pulmonary edema
            ▸ Dyspnea
            ▸ Orthopnea
            ▸ Paroxysmal nocturnal dyspnea
        (b) Tachycardia
        (c) ± chest pain
        (d) ± nausea and vomiting
        (e) ± diaphoresis
        (f) **Systolic murmur at the apex.**
        (g) S_2 is widely split
        (h) S_3 and S_4 audible
    (2) Laboratory
        (a) Chest X-ray
            Normal heart size with pulmonary edema.
        (b) ECG
            Sinus tachycardia
        (c) Echocardiography
            Valvular abnormalities
c. TREATMENT
    (1) Surgery
        Immediate surgery following preload and afterload reduction.

VII. INFECTIONS
    A. *Infective Endocarditis*
        1. DEFINITION
            a. An infection of the endocardium or valves of the heart.
            b. **Acute bacterial endocarditis is a medical emergency.**
            c. The infection may be acute or subacute
            d. Predisposing factors
                 (1) Rheumatic heart disease
                 (2) Congenital heart disease
                 (3) Degenerative valvular disease
                 (4) Mitral valve prolapse
                 (5) Injecting drug use
                 (6) Prosthetic valve

e. Etiologic categories of infective endocarditis
   (1) > 90% of endocarditis is caused by *Streptococci* spp., *Staphylococci* spp., and Enterococci sp.
   (2) Native valve endocarditis
       (a) *Streptococcus viridans*
       (b) Enterococci sp.
       (c) Other *Streptococci* sp.
       (d) *Staphylococcus aureus*
   (3) Right-sided endocarditis
       (a) Most commonly seen in injecting drug users, infected pacing wires and infected IV catheters.
       (b) Etiologies
           ‣ *Staphylococcus aureus*
           ‣ *Streptococci* spp.
           ‣ Enterococci sp.
   (4) Prosthetic valve endocarditis
       (a) ↑ risk of valve dehiscence and valve ring infection
       (b) Etiologies
           ‣ *Staphylococcus epidermidis*
           ‣ *Staphylococcus aureus*
           ‣ Gram-negative bacilli
           ‣ *Streptococcus viridans*

2. DIAGNOSIS
   a. Acute native valve endocarditis
      (1) Signs and symptoms
          (a) **The hallmark of infective endocarditis are regurgitant valvular murmurs.**
          (b) ↑ fever and chills
          (c) ± symptoms of heart failure
              ‣ Left-sided
                  • Symptoms of *acute* aortic or mitral regurgitation
                      ○ Pulmonary vascular congestion
                          · Dyspnea
                          · Orthopnea
                          · Paroxysmal nocturnal dyspnea
              ‣ Right-sided
                  • Heart failure less likely
                  • Tricuspid valve is most commonly involved
                      ○ Symptoms secondary to septic emboli
                          · Pleuritic chest pain

· Dyspnea
· Cough ± bloody sputum
(d) Physical findings secondary to embolization
- Renal
    CVA tenderness
- Splenic
    • Left upper quadrant pain ± radiation to left shoulder
    • Friction rub ± left pleural effusion
- CNS
    • Headache
    • Seizure
    • Encephalopathy
- Cardiac
    Chest pain
(2) Laboratory
(a) Leukocytosis ± left shift
(b) ± hematuria
(c) + blood cultures
    Usually x3 over 24 hours
(d) Chest X-ray
- Left-sided valvular involvement
    Pulmonary vascular redistribution
- Right-sided valvular involvement
    • Embolic abscesses
    • Pneumonia
(e) Echocardiography
    It can identify lesions but can't differentiate between active and healed valvular lesions.
b. Subacute native valve endocarditis
(1) Signs and symptoms
(a) **The hallmark of infective endocarditis are regurgitant valvular murmurs.**
(b) Fatigue
(c) ± fever/chills
(d) Diaphoresis
(e) Anorexia
(f) Night sweats
(g) Weight loss
(h) Arthralgias
(i) Clubbing

(j) Pallor

(k) Wasting

(2) Physical findings secondary to embolization

    (a) Renal

        CVA tenderness

    (b) Splenic

        ‣ Left upper quadrant pain ± radiation to left shoulder

        ‣ Friction rub ± left pleural effusion

    (c) CNS

        ‣ Headache

        ‣ Seizure

        ‣ Encephalopathy

    (d) Cardiac

        Chest pain

    (e) Peripheral manifestations secondary to vasculitis or emboli

        ‣ **Petechiae**

            On the hands, feet, conjunctiva and buccal mucosa

        ‣ **Roth spots**

            Hemorrhagic spots with a central pale area seen on fundoscopic exam

        ‣ **Janeway lesions**

            Painless erythematous nodules on the palms or soles

        ‣ **Splinter hemorrhages**

            Found under the nails

        ‣ **Osler's nodes**

            Reddish →purple nodules on the pads of fingers or toes that hurt

(3) Laboratory

    (a) Blood cultures

        ± x3 over 24 hours

    (b) Anemia

    (c) ↑ sedimentation rate

    (d) ↑ serum globulin level

    (e) + rheumatoid factor

    (f) Urinalysis

        ‣ Proteinuria

        ‣ Hematuria

    (g) Echocardiography

        It can identify lesions but can't differentiate between active and healed valvular lesions.

(h) Chest X-ray

± diagnosis of underlying valvular heart disease

3. TREATMENT

a. Identify organism and treat with appropriate antibiotics for 4 to 6 weeks.

b. Surgery may be needed to correct chronic valvular disease.

B. PERICARDIAL DISEASE

1. *Acute pericarditis*

a. DEFINITION

(1) An inflammation of the pericardium ± effusion.

(2) Most common etiologies

(a) **Idiopathic**

(b) Infectious

‣ *Viral*

‣ Bacterial

‣ Fungal

‣ Mycobacterial

‣ Parasitic

(c) Metastatic cancers

‣ Breast

‣ Lung

(d) Connective tissue diseases

‣ Rheumatic fever

‣ SLE

‣ Rheumatoid arthritis

(e) Chronic renal failure

(f) Drug reactions

‣ Procainamide

‣ Hydralazine

(g) Dressler's syndrome

(h) Radiation

(i) Trauma

b. DIAGNOSIS

(1) Signs and symptoms

(a) **A pericardial friction rub**

(b) Fever/chills

(c) Sharp, severe chest pain (better sitting up, leaning forward)

(d) Splinted breathing

(e) Anxiety

    (2) Laboratory
      (a) ECG
        ▸ PR depression
        ▸ Diffusely elevated ST
        ▸ Flattening of T waves
      (b) Chest X-ray
        ↑ cardiac silhouette if pericardial effusion is present
      (c) Echocardiography
        Sensitive enough to detect small amounts of fluid and pericardial thickening.
      (d) Infectious etiology
        ▸ ↑ ESR
        ▸ Leukocytosis
      (e) Allergic etiology
        Eosinophilia
      (f) Connective-tissue diseases
        ▸ + ANA
        ▸ + rheumatoid factor
      (g) Biopsy
        + In neoplasia, bacterial infection or mycobacterial infection
  c. TREATMENT
    (1) ASA or NSAIDs
    (2) Treatment of underlying disorder
    (3) Failure of therapy
      (a) Surgery
        Pericardiectomy
2. *Cardiac tamponade*
  a. DEFINITION
    (1) An accumulation of pericardial fluid, *under pressure* causing ↑ cardiac compression and ↓ cardiac output.
    (2) **This is a life-threatening emergency.**
  b. DIAGNOSIS
    (1) Signs and symptoms
      (a) Hypotension
      (b) Tachycardia
      (c) Dyspnea
      (d) Fatigue
      (e) Dizziness
      (f) Jugular vein distention
      (g) Pulsus paradoxus

(h) Pericardial friction rub

(i) ↑ area of cardiac dullness

(2) Laboratory

    (a) ECG

        ▸ PR depression,

        ▸ Nonspecific ST-T wave abnormalities

        ▸ **Electrical alterans**

            Alternation of every other P wave or QRS in height.

    (b) Chest X-ray

        >250 ccs of pericardial fluid will produce ↑ of cardiac shadow.

    (c) Echocardiogram

        ▸ Swinging motion of the heart within the pericardium

        ▸ Compression of the right ventricle and right atrium.

c. TREATMENT

  (1) Pericardiocentesis

  (2) IV fluids

  (3) Treatment of the underlying disorder

  (4) Surgery

    (a) Pericardiectomy

    (b) Pericardial window

3. *Constrictive pericarditis*

  a. DEFINITION

  Following a chronic inflammatory response, the pericardium becomes less flexible, thickens and sticks to the heart.

  b. DIAGNOSIS

    (1) Signs and symptoms

      (a) Fatigue

      (b) Dyspnea

      (c) Pulmonary congestion

      (d) Peripheral edema

      (e) Hepatomegaly

      (f) Ascites

      (g) Pericardial knock

      (h) Jugular vein distention

    (2) Laboratory

      (a) ECG

         ▸ Low voltage QRS

         ▸ Nonspecific T waves

      (b) Chest X-ray

         ▸ Pericardial calcification ≈ 50% of the time.

(c) Echocardiography
↑ thickness of pericardium with normal ventricular contraction.

   c. TREATMENT
      Pericardiectomy

VIII. CARDIOMYOPATHY
  A. *Dilated (Congestive) Cardiomyopathy*
    1. DEFINITION
      a. Failure of left ventricular contractility + dilatation of the ventricle.
      b. Etiologies
         (1) **Idiopathic**
         (2) Toxic
            (a) **ETOH**
            (b) Cancer chemotherapeutics
            (c) Heavy metals (cobalt)
         (3) Infectious
            (a) **Viral**
            (b) Bacterial
            (c) Parasitic
            (d) Tuberculosis
            (e) Rickettsial
            (f) Spirochetal
         (4) Collagen vascular diseases
         (5) Muscular dystrophy
         (6) Beriberi (Thiamine deficiency)
    2. DIAGNOSIS
      a. Relatively young patient + cardiac enlargement ± CHF ± systemic emboli ± ventricular arrhythmia ± chest pain.
      b. History
         Signs and symptoms of CHF and fatigue
      c. Physical exam
         (1) Enlarged heart
         (2) Gallop rhythm
         (3) Pulmonary congestion
         (4) Jugular vein distention
         (5) Mitral and tricuspid regurgitation
      d. Laboratory
         (1) ECG
            Nonspecific ST-T wave changes

(2) Chest X-ray

Cardiomegaly and signs of pulmonary congestion ± pleural effusion

(3) Echocardiography

Dilated ventricles + ↓ contraction

(4) Angiography

↓ stroke volume and cardiac output

3. TREATMENT

a. Treat the heart failure

b. Anticoagulation

c. Antiarrhythmics

d. Transplantation

4. COMPLICATIONS

a. ↓ cardiac output

b. Systemic embolization

c. Sudden death from ventricular arrhythmia

B. *Hypertrophic Cardiomyopathy*

1. DEFINITION

a. A marked left ventricular hypertrophy.

(1) 75% of patients have the nonobstructed form

(2) 25% of patients have the obstructive form

(a) Idiopathic hypertrophic subaortic stenosis

(b) Asymmetric septal hypertrophy

2. DIAGNOSIS

a. History

(1) Dyspnea on exertion

(2) Angina

(3) Syncope

b. Physical

(1) S_4

(2) Blowing murmur of mitral regurgitation at apex

(3) Harsh systolic murmur at the left sternal border

(4) Carotid pulse may be bisferiens in configuration or have a rapid upstroke

c. Laboratory

(1) ECG

Left ventricular hypertrophy

(2) Chest X-ray

Left ventricular hypertrophy

(3) Echocardiography

(a) IHSS

► Disproportionate septal thickening.

▸ Abnormalities of the aortic and mitral valves.
    (b) ASH
          ▸Disproportionate septal thickening.

3. TREATMENT
    a. Beta blockers or verapamil
    b. **Diuretics should be used cautiously**
    c. **Nitrates, digitalis and vasodilators are contraindicated.**
    d. Treatment of any arrhythmias
    e. Antibiotic prophylaxis for any valvular disease
    f. Surgical myectomy

4. COMPLICATIONS
    a. Systemic embolization
    b. Sudden death from ventricular arrhythmia

C. *Restrictive Cardiomyopathy*
  1. DEFINITION
    a. A disease characterized by ↓ ventricular filling during diastole secondary to ↑ myocardial stiffness.
    b. Etiologies
        (1) **Idiopathic**
        (2) Sarcoidosis
        (3) Amyloidosis
        (4) Hemochromatosis
        (5) Glycogen storage diseases
        (6) Cancer
            (a) Carcinoid
            (b) Metastatic
        (7) Radiation

  2. DIAGNOSIS
    a. Signs and symptoms
        (1) Abnormal diastolic ventricular filing
        (2) Varying degrees of systolic dysfunction
        (3) Expression of the underlying disease
    b. Laboratory
        (1) Studies to document underlying disease.
        (2) ECG
           Conduction defects
        (3) Echocardiography
            ▸ ↑ wall thickness
            ▸ Normal ventricular cavity
            ▸ ↓ contractility.

(4) Chest X-ray
> ► Pulmonary venous congestion with ± pleural effusion.

3. TREATMENT
    a. Treat the underlying illness
    b. Anticoagulation
    c. Antiarrhythmics
    d. Transplantation
4. COMPLICATIONS
    a. ↓ cardiac output
    b. Systemic embolization
    c. Sudden death from ventricular arrhythmia

IX. ACUTE RHEUMATIC FEVER
  A. DEFINITION

An *immunopathologic process* that can involve the heart, joints, skin and central nervous system following a group A beta-hemolytic streptococcal upper respiratory tract infection.

  B. DIAGNOSIS
    1. Modified Jones criteria
        a. Two major or one major and two minor manifestations *PLUS* evidence of *preceding* streptococcal infection.
        b. **Major Manifestations**
            (1) Carditis
            (2) Polyarthritis
            (3) Chorea
            (4) Erythema marginatum
            (5) Subcutaneous nodules
        c. **Minor Manifestations**
            (1) Fever ≥39°C. (102.2°F)
            (2) Arthralgias
            (3) Previous rheumatic fever
            (4) ↑ sedimentation rate or + C-reactive protein
            (5) Prolonged PR interval
        d. **Evidence of preceding group A Streptococcal infection**
            (1) + throat culture
            (2) History of scarlet fever
            (3) ↑ antistreptolysin O titer
            (4) Other + streptococcal antibodies
    2. Laboratory
        a. Leukocytosis
        b. ↑ sedimentation rate

        c. ↑ C-reactive protein

        d. Prolonged PR interval

C. TREATMENT

  1. Antibiotic therapy

    a. Doesn't change the course of acute rheumatic disease but a 10 day course of penicillin is given to eradicate any remaining streptococci.

      (1) Children weighing <60 pounds 600,000 units of benzathine penicillin G IM.

      (2) All patients >60 pounds 1,200,000 units of benzathine penicillin G IM.

      (3) Penicillin allergy, use erythromycin estolate 20-40 mg/kg in divided doses.

  2. Arthritis

    Aspirin is the mainstay of treatment

  3. Carditis

    a. Mild to moderate

      Aspirin for 2-6 weeks

    b. Severe

      (1) Systemic steroids

        (a) Prednisone for two weeks, then tapered for another two weeks

        (b) Then aspirin for 6-8 additional weeks

    c. Response to therapy measured by serial C-reactive protein levels

    d. Bed rest if CHF is diagnosed, bed rest until it resolves

  4. Chorea

    a. Quiet environment

    b. Sedatives

    c. ± phenobarbital

    d. ± haloperidol

D. PROPHYLAXIS

  1. Weight >27 kg = Benzathine penicillin G 1.2 million units IM every 3-4 weeks or

  2. Weight <27 kg = Benzathine penicillin G 600,000 million units IM every 3-4 weeks or

  3. Erythromycin 250 mg or sulfadiazine 500 mg in children <30 kg or 1 g. in adults PO daily

  4. **Always premedicate before any surgical, dental or invasive diagnostic procedures if valvular disease is present.**

    a. Dental and upper respiratory tract surgery

      (1) One hour before and half the dose 6 hours after

        (a) Amoxicillin

          ▸ <15 kg.........750 mg

          ▸ 15-30 kg....1500 mg

          ▸ >30 kg.......3000 mg

        (b) Erythromycin succinate (For PCN allergy)

          ▸ <30 kg......20 mg/kg

          ▸ >30 kg.......1000 mg

I. ESOPHAGUS
A. *Dysphagia*
1. Difficulty swallowing
   a. Oropharyngeal dysphagia
      "Transfer dysphagia". Difficulty *transferring* the food bolus into the upper esophagus.
   b. Esophageal dysphagia
      Difficulty moving the food bolus from the upper esophagus to the stomach.
2. Most common etiologies
   a. Oropharyngeal (Pre-esophageal)
      (1) Local structural lesions
         (a) Carcinoma
         (b) Zenker's diverticulum
         (c) **Plummer-Vinson syndrome**
            In females, iron deficiency anemia + esophageal webbing
      (2) **Neuromuscular diseases ≈80% of cases**
         (a) MS
         (b) Myasthenia gravis
         (c) Parkinson's disease
         (d) Stroke
      (3) Upper esophageal sphincter dysfunction
   b. Esophageal
      (1) Strictures
         (a) Peptic
         (b) Chemical
      (2) Carcinoma
      (3) Barrett's esophagus
         (a) Metaplastic columnar epithelium replaces normal squamous epithelium.
         (b)↑ risk of malignant transformation
      (4) Schatski ring
      (5) Achalasia
B. *Gastroesophageal Reflux Disease*
1. DEFINITION
   Reflux of gastric contents into the esophagus usually causing esophageal inflammation
2. DIAGNOSIS
   a. History and Physical
      (1) Odynophagia (Painful swallowing)
      (2) Pyrosis (Heartburn)

   (3) Regurgitation

   (4) Chest pain

   (5) Dysphagia

  b. Laboratory

   (1) Barium swallow

    (a) Although it can identify reflux, it is unreliable

    (b) It can identify strictures

   (2) Endoscopy

    Direct observation of mucosa ± biopsies

   (3) 24 hour esophageal luminal pH recording

 3. TREATMENT

  a. Nonpharmacologic

   (1) Elevate the head of the bed

   (2) Avoid late night meals or snacks

   (3) ↓ cigarettes, caffeine and ETOH

   (4) ↓ fats

   (5) Weight loss

  b. Pharmacologic

   (1) Antacids

   (2) H_2-receptor antagonists

   (3) Metoclopramide

   (4) Omeprazole

   (5) Cisapride

  c. Surgery

   (1) Belsey repair

   (2) Nissen fundoplication

C. *Esophageal Cancer*

 1. DEFINITION

  a. A primary malignancy of the esophagus

   (1) **Squamous cell carcinoma.....≈95%**

   (2) Adenocarcinoma......................≈5%

    (a) Gastroesophageal junction

    (b) Barrett's esophagus

  b. Location

   (1) Upper third.........≈10%

   (2) Middle third........≈40%

   (3) Lower third.........≈50%

 2. DIAGNOSIS

  a. History and Physical

   (1) **Dysphagia**

(2) Weight loss

(3) ± Pain

b. Laboratory

(1) Barium swallow → identification of esophageal lesion.

(2) Endoscopy + biopsy → diagnosis

(3) CT of the chest → staging

3. TREATMENT

a. Surgery

(1) Less than 10% 5-year survival.

(2) ↑ surgical mortality

b. Radiation

May be of some benefit in lesions of the upper third of the esophagus

c. Chemotherapy

Not useful

4. PROGNOSIS

Poor

II. STOMACH

A. *Peptic Ulcer Disease*

1. DEFINITION

a. A defect in the gastrointestinal mucosa which penetrates the muscularis mucosa.

b. Etiologies

(1) Genetic Predisposition

(2) ↑ acid secretion

(3) Direct injury to the mucosa

(a) Aspirin

(b) NSAID

(c) *Helicobacter pylori*

‣ Present in 90% of duodenal ulcers and 75% in gastric ulcers.

‣ Treatment ↓ recurrence of PUD by 75-90%

(4) ↓ bicarbonate

(a) Smoking

(b) Acidosis

(5) Stress? caffeine?

(6) Systemic disease

(a) Renal failure

(b) Chronic lung disease

c. **Duodenal ulcers are most common.**

d. Gastric ulcers are less common.

2. DIAGNOSIS
    a. History and Physical
        (1) Dyspepsia
            (a) Nausea
            (b) Vomiting
            (c) Anorexia
            (d) Epigastric fullness
            (e) Bloating
            (f) Pain
                ▸ Nocturnal
                ▸ Burning epigastric
            (g) Heartburn
            (h) Early satiety
            (i) Weight loss
    b. Laboratory
        (1) Upper GI
        (2) Endoscopy + biopsies of ulcer margins ± brush cytologies.
3. TREATMENT
    a. Nonpharmacologic
        (1) ↓ cigarettes
        (2) ↓ NSAID and aspirin
        (3) ↓ emotional stress
    b. Pharmacologic
        (1) Antacids
        (2) H_2-receptor antagonists
        (3) Sucralfate
        (4) Lansoprazole
        (5) Anxiolytics/antidepressants
        (6) Eradication of *Helicobacter pylori*
            (a) Tetracycline 500 mg or metronidazole 250 mg tid + bismuth tablets
            (b) Omeprazole + amoxicillin or clarithromycin
            (c) Ranitidine + metronidazole and amoxicillin
        (7) Maintenance therapy to prevent recurrences.
    c. Surgery
        (1) Subtotal gastrectomy
        (2) Truncal vagotomy and pyloroplasty
        (3) Truncal vagotomy and antrectomy
        (4) Proximal gastric vagotomy
4. COMPLICATIONS
    a. Hemorrhage

       b. Perforation

       c. Obstruction

B. *Cancer of the Stomach*

   1. DEFINITION

       a. A primary malignancy of the stomach

           (1) Adenocarcinomas........................$\approx$90%

           (2) Lymphomas, leiomyosarcomas......$\approx$10%

       b. Location

           (1) Pylorus and antrum....................$\approx$**50%**

           (2) Lesser curvature.........................$\approx$20%

           (3) Body...$\approx$20%

           (4) Cardia......................................$\approx$ 7%

           (5) Greater curvature.........................$\approx$ 3%

   2. DIAGNOSIS

       a. Early gastric carcinomas are frequently silent.

       b. History (as the disease progresses)

           (1) Anorexia

           (2) Pain

           (3) Weight loss

           (4) Vomiting

       c. Physical

           (1) There are no physical findings in early disease.

           (2) Physical findings in advanced disease are all related to metastases.

       d. Laboratory

           (1) Upper GI

               Identification of a stomach lesion which may or may not be suggestive of a malignancy.

           (2) Endoscopy + biopsy $\rightarrow$ diagnosis

   3. TREATMENT

       a. < 33% of tumors are resectable for cure at presentation

       b. Surgery

           (1) Curative resection

           (2) Palliative resection

       c. Radiation therapy

           Gastric carcinoma is relatively radioresistant

       d. Chemotherapy

           Multiple agents have extended survival time.

   4. PROGNOSIS

       a. Five-year survival

           For most patients is <5%.

III. SMALL AND LARGE BOWEL
A. Inflammatory Bowel Disease
1. *Ulcerative Colitis*
a. DEFINITION
(1) An inflammatory bowel disease characterized by *superficial inflammation* of the colonic mucosa.
(2) The inflammation begins at the rectum and moves proximally.
(3) The inflammation is diffuse and continuous
b. DIAGNOSIS
(1) History and Physical
(a) Rectal bleeding
(b) **Bloody diarrhea**
(c) Tenesmus
(d) Abdominal cramping
(e) Weight loss
(f) Extraintestinal disease can occur affecting the skin, eyes, joints, and liver
(2) Laboratory
(a) Barium enema
  ‣ Tubular *ahaustral* segment of colon ± edema ± ulcerations
(b) **Colonoscopy and biopsy**
  ‣ Rectal involvement
  ‣ Mucosal erythema, ulcerations, hemorrhage and exudate.
  ‣ The mucosa is friable
  ‣ Crypt abscesses
c. TREATMENT
(1) Diet
(2) Antidiarrheal and anticholinergics in mild/moderate disease only
(3) Oral anti-inflammatories
(a) Sulfasalazine
(b) 5-ASA preparations
  ‣ Olsalazine
  ‣ Mesalamine
(4) Topical anti-inflammatories
(a) Mesalamine enemas
(b) Steroid enemas
(5) Corticosteroids
Prednisone
(6) Immunosuppressive agents
(a) Azothioprine

     (b) 6-mercaptopurine

   (7) Surgery

     Colectomy for intractable disease

  d. COMPLICATIONS

   (1) Perforation

   (2) Toxic Megacolon

   (3) Stricture

   (4) ↑ **risk of colon cancer.**

 2. *Crohn's Disease*

  a. DEFINITION

   (1) An inflammatory bowel disease characterized by *transmural inflammation.*

   (2) The inflammation can occur from the mouth to the anus

    Ileum and right colon are most common

   (3) The inflammation is focal and asymmetric

   (4) Noncaseating granulomas are present

   (5) Extraintestinal disease can occur affecting the skin, eyes, joints, and liver

  b. DIAGNOSIS

   (1) History and Physical findings are dependent upon location and severity of inflammation.

    (a) General

     ‣ Weight loss

     ‣ Fever and/or night sweats

     ‣ Fatigue

    (b) Stomach

     ‣ Epigastric pain

     ‣ Nausea and vomiting

    (c) Intestinal

     ‣ Abdominal pain

     ‣ Cramping

    (d) Colon

     ‣ Abdominal pain

     ‣ Rectal bleeding

     ‣ Nonbloody diarrhea

   (2) Laboratory

    (a) Endoscopic findings

     ‣ Cobble stoning

     ‣ Linear ulcers

     ‣ Discontinuous involvement

    (b) Barium enema

     ‣ Discontinuous involvement

▸ Classic "string sign"

c. TREATMENT
   (1) Diet
   (2) Antidiarrheal and anticholinergics in mild/moderate disease only
   (3) Oral anti-inflammatories
      (a) Sulfasalazine
      (b) 5-ASA preparations
         ▸ Olsalazine
         ▸ Mesalamine
   (4) Topical anti-inflammatories
      (a) Mesalamine enemas
      (b) Steroid enemas
   (5) Metronidazole
   (6) Corticosteroids
      Prednisone
   (7) Immunosuppressive agents
      (a) Azothioprine
      (b) 6-mercaptopurine
   (8) Antibiotics (to treat microabscesses)
      (a) Tetracycline
      (b) Amoxicillin
      (c) Ciprofloxacin
      (d) Trimethoprim-sulfamethoxazole
   (9) Surgery for intractable disease
d. COMPLICATIONS
   (1) Fistulas
   (2) Intestinal obstruction
   (3) Strictures
   (4) Abscess
   (5) ↑ **risk of colon cancer.**

B. DIVERTICULAR DISEASE
   1. *Diverticulosis*
   a. DEFINITION
      (1) The presence of diverticula in the colon
         (a) Not true diverticula but herniations of mucosa and submucosa through the muscularis.
         (b) Most are in the sigmoid colon
      (2) The etiology is unknown

b. DIAGNOSIS
 (1) History and Physical
  (a) Usually asymptomatic
  (b) LLQ pain
  (c) Changes in bowel habit
  (d) ± rectal bleeding
 (2) Laboratory
  (a) Barium enema
   Identifies diverticula
c. TREATMENT
 (1) ↑ fiber
 (2) Antispasmodics

2. *Diverticulitis*
 a. DEFINITION
  (1) Microperforation of a diverticula secondary to inspissated feces
  (2) The most common complication of diverticulosis.
  (3) 90% of cases involve the sigmoid colon.
 b. DIAGNOSIS
  (1) History and Physical
   (a) Fever
   (b) LLQ pain
    ▸ ± guarding
    ▸ ± rebound
   (c) Nausea and vomiting
   (d) Change in bowel habit
   (e) ↓ bowel sounds
  (2) Laboratory
   (a) ↑ WBC count
   (b) Barium enema
   (c) CT of the abdomen if there is a question of diagnosis
 c. TREATMENT
  (1) Mild/moderate disease
   (a) NPO → Clear fluids → Soft diet → High fiber diet
   (b) Pain medication
    No opiates
   (c) Antibiotics
    ▸ Amoxicillin
    ▸ Amoxicillin + metronidazole
    ▸ Tetracycline

           (2) Severe disease

               (a) Hospitalization

               (b) IV fluids

               (c) IV antibiotics

                    ▸ Gentamycin + clindamycin

                    ▸ Cefoxin

                    ▸ Imipenem

               (d) Surgery

       d. COMPLICATIONS

           (1) Hemorrhage

           (2) Perforation

           (3) Pericolic abscess

           (4) Peritonitis

           (5) Fistula

           (6) Stricture

D. *Colonic Polyps*

   1 General

       a. Three types of polyps can arise in the colon

           (1) Hyperplastic

               (a) Small polyps usually <5 mm.

               (b) Little to no malignant potential

           (2) Inflammatory

           (3) Adenomatous (Neoplastic)

               (a) Tubular......................≈60%

               (b) Tubulovillous.........≈20-30%

               (c) Villous........................≈10%

       b. The majority of polyps are *hyperplastic*

       c. The majority of polyps are <1 cm.

       d. Risk of malignant transformation

           (1) ↑ with size

               (a) <1 cm............................≈1%

               (b) 1-2 cm.........................≈10%

               (c) >2 cm....................≈30-50%

           (2) Polyp type

               (a) Tubular...........................-5%

               (b) Tubulovillous............≈5-20%

               (c) Villous adenoma......≈30-70%

           (3) ↑ numbers of polyps ↑ the risk

       e. Treatment

       Removal of the polyps upon or shortly after diagnosis.

E. *Colonic Cancer*
1. DEFINITION
   a. A primary malignancy arising from the colonic mucosa.
   b. **98% are adenocarcinoma above the anal verge.**
   c. 80% are below the middle portion of the descending colon
2. DIAGNOSIS
   a. History and Physical
      (1) Left colon
         (a) **Rectal bleeding**
         (b) **Change in bowel habit**
         (c) Tenesmus
         (d) Pencil stools
         (e) Vague abdominal or back pain
      (2) Right colon
         (a) Guaiac + stools
         (b) RLQ pain
         (c) Weight loss
      (3) ≈33% of patients will present with metastasis
   b. Laboratory
      (1) CBC
         Iron deficiency anemia
      (2) + occult blood
      (3) ↑ CEA (not specific)
      (4) Liver scan
         If ↑ liver function studies or hepatomegaly
      (5) Bone scan
         If ↑ of alkaline phosphatase or bone pain
      (6) Barium Enema
         Can detect cancer >90% of cases
      (7) Colonoscopy with biopsy
         Has almost 100% rate of establishing diagnosis
      (8) CT scan
         Preoperatively to exclude synchronous lesions and metastatic disease
3. TREATMENT
   a. Surgery
      (1) Dependent upon location of tumor
         (a) Right- or left-sided lesions
            Hemicolectomy
         (b) Upper rectum, sigmoid
            Anterior resection with anastomosis to the rectal stump

(c) Distal lesions of the rectum

Abdominal-Perineal resection with permanent colostomy

(2) Palliative surgery for metastatic disease to control obstruction, bleeding or perforation

b. Radiation

(1) Pre- or postoperative radiation of rectal lesions to prevent local recurrence.

(2) Treatment of advanced disease to alleviate obstruction and bony pain

c. Chemotherapy

↑ survival for Duke's C with combination 5-fluorouracil + levamisole

4. PROGNOSIS

a. Duke's A.............................>80%

b. Duke's B........................≈60-80%

c. Duke's C.............................≈50%

d. Duke's D.............................<25%

e. The ↑ in the penetration of the wall of the colon, the ↓ the prognosis.

IV. GALLBLADDER

A. *Acute Cholecystitis*

1. DEFINITION

a. An acute inflammation of the gallbladder

(1) Etiologies

(a) **95% calculous**

(b) 5% acalculous

2. DIAGNOSIS

a. History and Physical

(1) RUQ or epigastric pain

(2) Nausea and vomiting

(3) Anorexia

(4) Low-grade fever

(5) Murphy's sign

"Classic" physical finding in which there is inspiratory arrest during deep palpation of the right upper quadrant

b. Laboratory

(1) ↑ WBC count

(2) ± abnormal liver function studies

(3) **Abdominal ultrasound**

(a) Gallstones

(b) ↑ edema/thickness gallbladder wall

(c) Distention

3. TREATMENT
   a. Hospitalization
   b. NPO
   c. IV fluids
   d. Pain medication
   e. Antibiotics
      (1) Ampicillin
      (2) Cephalosporins
   f. Surgery following improvement
4. COMPLICATIONS
   a. Empyema
   b. Perforation
      (1) Pericholecystic abscess
      (2) Peritonitis
   c. Fistula
B. *Chronic Cholecystitis*
   1. DEFINITION
      a. An inflammation of the gallbladder secondary to gallstones
      b. Characterized by *recurrent* attacks of RUQ pain secondary to *transient* obstruction of the cystic duct by gallstones.
   2. DIAGNOSIS
      a. History and Physical
         (1) Postprandial RUQ or epigastric pain and tenderness
         (2) Nausea and vomiting
         (3) Belching
         (4) Bloating
         (5) Fatty food intolerance
      b. Laboratory
         (1) **Abdominal ultrasound**
            (a) + for gallstones
            (b) ↑ thickness wall and a contracted gallbladder
   3. TREATMENT
      Surgery
C. *Cholelithiasis*
   1. DEFINITION
      a. The formation of "stones" within the gallbladder
      b. Stone analysis
         (1) Cholesterol/mixed stones..........≈80%
         (2) Pigmented stones.....................≈20%

c. Etiologies
(1) The four "F"
(a) Fat
(b) Forty
(c) Female
(d) Fertile
(2) Oral contraceptive use
(3) Pregnancy
(4) Diabetes
(5) Hyperlipidemia, type IV
2. DIAGNOSIS
a. History and Physical
(1) May be asymptomatic
(2) RUQ and/or epigastric pain following meals
(3) Nausea and vomiting
b. Laboratory
(1) **Abdominal ultrasound**
+ for gallstones
3. TREATMENT
Surgery

V. **LIVER**
A. Viral Hepatitis
1. *Hepatitis A*
a. DEFINITION
(1) An infection of the liver caused by a 27 nm RNA virus that attacks the hepatocytes in the liver.
(2) Transmission
(a) **Fecal-oral**
Water/food-borne contamination
(b) Sexual
(c) Blood
(3) Incubation
(a) 2-6 weeks
(b) Greatest infectivity the two weeks *before* clinical illness.
(4) **No chronic form or carrier state**
(5) Fulminant disease is rare

b. DIAGNOSIS

    (1) History and Physical

        (a) Mild disease

            Subclinical or flu-like symptoms

        (b) Moderate

            ‣ Fatigue

            ‣ Malaise

            ‣ Fever

            ‣ Anorexia

            ‣ Alteration in taste and small

            ‣ Nausea and vomiting

            ‣ RUQ pain or discomfort

            ‣ ± jaundice

            ‣ Dark urine

    (2) Laboratory

        (a) Abnormal liver function studies

            ‣ ↑ GGTP

            ‣ ↑ AST

            ‣ ↑ ALT

            ‣ ± ↑ bilirubin

            ‣ Moderate ↑ of alkaline phosphatase

        (b) Serologies

            ‣ Anti-HAV IgM

                Current or recent infection or convalescence

            ‣ Anti-HAV IgG

                Recovered or vaccination.

c. TREATMENT

    (1) Supportive care

    (2) Antiemetics

    (3) Monitor liver function

    (4) Alcohol should be avoided

    (5) Corticosteroids have no place in the treatment of acute viral hepatitis

d. PROPHYLAXIS

    (1) Treat contacts with immune serum globulin

    (2) Hepatitis A vaccine for *active immunization* for patients ≥ 2 years of age.

e. PROGNOSIS

    Excellent

2. *Hepatitis B*
    a. DEFINITION
        (1) An infection of the liver caused by a 42 nm DNA virus that attacks the hepatocytes in the liver.
        (2) Transmission
            (a) Parenteral contact
                ‣ Needle stick/transfusion
                ‣ Sexual contact
                ‣ Perinatal transmission
            (b) Hepatitis B is present in blood for a protracted period of time.
        (3) Carrier state can occur
            (a) Persistent circulating viral particles
            (b) No histologic evidence of hepatic inflammation
            (c) Normal liver function studies
        (4) Chronic hepatitis can occur
        (5) Fulminant disease <5%
        (6) Incubation
            4 weeks to 6 months
        (7) Hepatitis B antigens
            (a) HBsAg
                ‣ Surface antigen present before the onset of clinical illness and persists through early convalescence.
                ‣ Persistence of circulating HBsAg may indicate progression to chronic hepatitis B.
            (b) HBcAg
                ‣ Nucleocapsid core does not freely circulate
                ‣ Found in hepatocytes when there is *active* viral replication
            (c) HBeAg
                ‣ HBcAg *circulating form*
                ‣ A marker of active viral replication and infectivity
                ‣ Persistence of circulating HbeAg > 3-4 months indicates likely progression to chronic hepatitis B.
    b. DIAGNOSIS
        (1) History and Physical
            (a) Fatigue
            (b) ± fever
            (c) Nausea ± vomiting
            (d) Jaundice
            (e) Dark urine

(f) Immune complex disease
- ▸ Urticaria
- ▸ Arthritis
- ▸ Arthralgias
- ▸ Glomerulonephritis
- ▸ Vasculitis

(g) Fulminant hepatitis
- ▸ Liver failure
- ▸ Coagulopathy
- ▸ Encephalopathy

(2) Laboratory

(a) Abnormal liver function studies
- ▸ ↑ GGTP
- ▸ ↑ AST
- ▸ ↑ ALT
- ▸ ± ↑ bilirubin
- ▸ Moderate ↑ of alkaline phosphatase

(b) Serologies
- ▸ Anti-HBs
  - • Antibody to surface antigen
  - • Appears following hepatitis B infection or vaccination
  - • **Confers immunity and is protective**
- ▸ Anti-HBc
  - • Antibodies to HBV core antigen
    - ◦ Anti-HBc IgM
      - · + during acute hepatitis B infection
      - · ± during chronic hepatitis B infection
    - ◦ Anti-HBcTotal
      - · ↑ in acute infection
        - ↑ anti-HBc IgM
      - · ↑ in chronic infection
        - ↑ anti-HBc IgG
      - · ↑ in patients who have recovered
  - • Usually as infection resolves there is ↓ levels of anti-Hbc IgM and ↑ levels of anti-HBc IgG
- ▸ HbeAg
  - • Correlates to viral replication in the liver
  - • Appears early in acute infection and disappears in a few weeks

• Persistence > 3-4 months usually progression to chronic hepatitis B

    (c) Liver biopsy

      ▸ Histologic diagnosis for chronic persistent or chronic active hepatitis

        • **Chronic persistent hepatitis**

          ○ Mononuclear cell infiltrate limited to portal tracts

          ○ Usually nonprogressive

          ○ Cirrhosis is rare

        • **Chronic active hepatitis**

          ○ Piecemeal necrosis

            · Mononuclear cell infiltrate that extends past the portal tracts and into the peri-portal space

          ○ Progressive

          ○ Cirrhosis is more common

          ○ ↑ incidence of hepatocellular carcinoma

  (3) Chronic hepatitis B

    (a) Criteria for diagnosis

      ▸ Clinical evidence of HBV infection ≥ 6 months

      ▸ Abnormal liver function studies

      ▸ Documented histologic findings of ongoing hepatic infection

    (b) Likelihood in developing chronic hepatitis B is ≈5-10%.

    (c) Serologies

      ▸ + HbsAg

      ▸ ↑ levels of Anti-HBcTotal

    (d) The prognosis for chronic hepatitis B is variable

c. TREATMENT

  (1) Supportive care

  (2) Antiemetics

  (3) Monitor liver function

  (4) Alcohol should be avoided

  (5) Corticosteroids have no place in the treatment of acute viral hepatitis

  (6) Interferon-alpha for chronic hepatitis B

d. PROPHYLAXIS

  (1) Unvaccinated patients exposed to HBV

    (a) Hepatitis B immune globulin

    (b) HBV vaccine

(2) Previously vaccinated

Test for anti-HBs and if the titer is < 10 ml U/mL. treat as above

4. *Hepatitis C*

a. DEFINITION

(1) An infection of the liver caused by an RNA virus that attacks the hepatocytes in the liver.

(2) Transmission

(a) Parenteral contact

▸ **The major cause of post-transfusion hepatitis.**

▸ Needle sticks or injecting drug use

Injecting drug use accounts for ≈50% of the cases

(b) Sexual

(c) Perinatal

(3) Incubation

2 weeks-6 months

(4) Carrier state exists

(5) Chronic hepatitis C

(a) ≈50-60% of acute hepatitis C progresses to chronic hepatitis C

(b) ↑ risk of cirrhosis

(c) ↑ risk of hepatocellular carcinoma

(6) Fulminant disease in <5% of cases

b. DIAGNOSIS

(1) History and Physical

(a) Acute hepatitis C is clinically silent in over 90% of patients

(2) Laboratory

(a) Liver function studies

Fluctuating ↑ levels of GGTP, AST and ALT

(b) Serologies

▸ Anti-HCV

• Second-generation enzyme radioimmunoassay

• + weeks to months after exposure

• Not protective

▸ Confirmation of Anti-HCV with RIBA-II

Recombinant immunoblot assay

(c) Liver biopsy in chronic disease

c. TREATMENT

(1) Supportive care

(2) Monitor liver function

(3) Interferon-alpha for chronic hepatitis C

(4) ? Immune serum globulin

5. *Hepatitis D*

    a. DEFINITION

        (1) An infection of the liver caused by an RNA virus or *delta agent* that attacks the hepatocytes in the liver.

        (2) **HBV infection must be present for infection to occur**.

            (a) Coinfection

                Simultaneous infection with both hepatitis B and hepatitis D

            (b) Superinfection

                ▸ Chronic hepatitis B infection when exposed to delta agent

                ▸ ↑ risk of cirrhosis

                ▸ ↑ risk of fulminant liver failure

        (3) Transmission

            (a) Blood

                ▸ In the United States and western Europe

                    • Injecting drug use

                    • Multiply transfused hemophiliacs

            (b) Sexual and perinatal

                South America, Middle East, Mediterranean basin

        (4) Incubation

            3 weeks-3 months

        (5) Carrier state exists

        (6) **Chronic hepatitis occurs in most patients**

        (7) Fulminant disease occurs ≈5-20% of patients

    b. DIAGNOSIS

        (1) History and physical

            See hepatitis B

        (2) Laboratory

            (a) Serologies

                ▸ Coinfection

                    • Anti-HDV IgM in ↓ titers or transiently present

                    • HDAg

                ▸ Superinfection

                    • Anti-HDV in ↑ sustained titers

                    • HDAg

    c. TREATMENT

        See hepatitis B

    d. PROPHYLAXIS

        None

6. *Hepatitis E*
   a. DEFINITION
      (1) An infection of the liver caused by an unclassified RNA virus that attacks the hepatocytes in the liver.
      (2) Transmission
         (a) Fecal-oral
         (b) Travelers to endemic areas are at risk.
         (c) No reported cases of hepatitis E acquired in the United States
      (3) Incubation
         15-60 days
      (4) Carrier state does not exist
      (5) Chronic hepatitis E does not occur
      (6) Fulminant disease 1-2% but 10-30% in pregnant women
   b. DIAGNOSIS
      (1) History and Physical
         Similar to hepatitis A
      (2) Laboratory
         (a) Serologies
            ▸ HEVAg and Anti-HEV assays available from the CDC
   c. TREATMENT
      See hepatitis A
   d. PROPHYLAXIS
      None
C. *Hepatic Carcinoma*
   1. DEFINITION
      a. A primary malignancy of the hepatic parenchyma.
         Hepatocellular (Hepatoma) ≈70-90% of cases
      b. A primary malignancy of the hepatic bile ducts
         Cholangiocarcinoma ≈10-30% of cases.
      c. Predisposing conditions
         (1) **Cirrhosis**
         (2) Chronic hepatitis B
         (3) Chronic hepatitis C
   2. DIAGNOSIS
      a. History and Physical
         (1) RUQ mass and tenderness
         (2) Abdominal pain
         (3) Weight loss
         (4) Nausea and vomiting
         (5) Ascites

b. Laboratory
    (1) Abnormal liver function studies
    (2) Alpha-fetoprotein
        + in ≈70% of cases but is not diagnostic
    (3) Ultrasound
        Excellent technique to screen for liver mass
    (4) MRI or CT
        Valuable to evaluate tumor and vascular invasion
    (5) **Biopsy is the definitive test for diagnosis**
3. TREATMENT
    a. Surgery
        Only for solitary hepatoma
    b. Radiation
        Low-dose radiation to alleviate liver pain
    c. Chemotherapy
        Hepatic artery perfusion
            ≈50% have a response and median survival↑ to over a year
    d. Liver transplantation
        Appropriate for selected patients
4. PROGNOSIS
    Median survival for all patients is ≈5 months

VI. **PANCREAS**
    A. *Acute Pancreatitis*
        1. DEFINITION
            a. An inflammation of the pancreas. The inflammation caused by pancreatic auto-digestion, can run the gamut from mild disease to life-threatening illness.
            b. Acute pancreatitis will usually resolve along with *normal* pancreatic function.
            c. Etiologies
                (1) **>80% secondary to gallstones or ETOH abuse**
                (2) ≈10% are idiopathic
                (3) Miscellaneous
                    (a) Trauma
                    (b) Hyperparathyroidism
                    (c) Hyperlipidemia
                    (d) Infection
        2. DIAGNOSIS
            a. History and Physical
                (1) ↑ pain, "boring" or "stabbing" in the LUQ or midepigastrium.
                (2) Nausea ± vomiting

        (3) Dehydration

        (4) Fever

        (5) Tachypnea

        (6) Tachycardia

        (7) $\updownarrow$ BP

        (8) Abdominal distention

        (9) $\downarrow$ bowel sounds

     (10) $\pm$ guarding

     (11) In severe disease

           (a) Shock

           (b) Hemorrhage (rare)

              ▸ Grey Turner sign

                  Large flank ecchymosis

              ▸ Cullen sign

                  Periumbilical ecchymosis

  b. Laboratory

        (1) $\uparrow$ serum amylase

        (2) $\uparrow$ serum lipase

        (3) Ultrasonography

           May detect gallstones, $\uparrow$ edema or enlargement of pancreas

        (4) CT of abdomen

           Confirms the diagnosis

3. TREATMENT

  a. Mild to moderate disease

        (1) Hospitalization

        (2) Correct dehydration

        (3) Monitor calcium levels

        (4) NPO

        (5) Nasogastric tube to alleviate nausea and vomiting

        (6) Pain control

        (7) H_2 receptor antagonists

        (8) Antibiotic therapy

           (a) For severe necrotizing pancreatitis

           (b) Adjunct during surgical intervention

  b. Severe

        (1) Admit ICU for treatment if any of the following present

           (a) Shock

           (b) Respiratory failure

           (c) Renal failure

(d) Severe metabolic complications
- ► Hyperglycemia
- ► Hypercalcemia

4. COMPLICATIONS
- a. Intra-abdominal infections (pancreatic phlegmon)
    - (1) Laparotomy with debridement/drainage
    - (2) C&S of fluid/debris and appropriate antibiotic therapy.
- b. Hemorrhage (rare)
    - Immediate laparotomy
- c. Pancreatic pseudocysts
    - (1) Diagnosed by ultrasound cured by surgery
        - (a) Complications
            - ► Rupture
            - ► Infection
            - ► Hemorrhage
- d. Pulmonary complications
    - Atelectasis → pneumonia → ARDS
- e. Acute renal failure

B. *Chronic Pancreatitis*
1. DEFINITION
- a. An inflammation of the pancreas caused by
    - Recurrent bouts of acute pancreatitis yielding replacement of the exocrine and endocrine pancreas by scar tissue
- b. Chronic pancreatitis will result in the *loss* of normal pancreatic function.
- c. Common Etiologies
    - (1) **ETOH abuse**
    - (2) Idiopathic (>25%)
    - (3) Trauma
    - (4) Hypercalcemia
    - (5) Cystic fibrosis

2. DIAGNOSIS
- a. History and Physical
    - (1) Abdominal pain
        - (a) Usually epigastric with referred pain to the back 50% of the time
        - (b) ↑ pain when eating
    - (2) Weight loss
    - (3) Steatorrhea
- b. Laboratory
    - (1) ± mild ↑ amylase or lipase
    - (2) ± mild ↑ liver function studies

(3) Abnormal bentiromide (Chymex) test

(4) Abnormal secretin stimulation test

(5) ↑ stool fats (quantitative)

(6) Plain films of the abdomen

    Pancreatic calcifications a third to half the time.

(7) Abdominal ultrasound

    Identify pseudocysts

(8) CT of abdomen

    (a) Identify pseudocysts

    (b) Identify dilation of main pancreatic duct

    (c) Rule out cancer of the pancreas

3. TREATMENT

    a. Pain control

    b. Control malabsorption

    c. Low fat diet

    d. Stop ETOH

    e. H_2-receptor antagonists

    f. Fat-soluble vitamin supplementation

    g. Correct the endocrine insufficiency

4. PROGNOSIS

    a. Ranson's criteria

    (1) On admission

        (a) > age 55

        (b) WBC > 16,000/mm³

        (c) Abnormal liver function studies

            ▸ LDH >350 IU/L

            ▸ SGOT >250 U/L

        (d) Blood glucose >200 mg/dL

    (2) Within 48 hours of admission

        (a) ↑ BUN >5 mg/dL

        (b) ↓ hematocrit by ≥10%

        (c) ≥6 L volume replacement

        (d) Base deficit >4 mEq/L

        (e) Serum calcium <8 mg/dL

        (f) PaO_2 <60 mm Hg

    (3) Morbidity and mortality

        (a) <3 criteria

            1% mortality

                    (b) 3-7 criteria
                            ‣ 50% require ICU admission
                            ‣ 15% mortality
                    (c) >7 criteria
                            ‣ 100% require ICU admission
                            ‣ 50% mortality

C. *Pancreatic Cancer*
   1. DEFINITION
      a. A primary malignancy of the exocrine pancreas.
      b. **≈90% are duct cell adenocarcinomas.**
         66% of the time these lesions are in the head of the pancreas
   2. DIAGNOSIS
      a. History and Physical
        (1) **Signs and symptoms of illness occur late in the course of disease.**
           (a) Weight loss
           (b) Pain
           (c) Jaundice
           (d) Anorexia
           (e) Hepatomegaly (late)
           (f) Epigastric mass (late)
      b. Laboratory
        (1) Lipase, amylase, and liver function studies may be abnormal but cannot distinguish cancer from pancreatitis.
        (2) Abdominal CT scan
           Diagnosis ≈90% of the time
        (3) (ERCP) Endoscopic retrograde cholangiopancreatography
           Diagnosis ≈90-95% of the time
   3. TREATMENT
      a. Surgery
        (1) ≈10% are resectable, of these 5-year survival is ≈10%.
        (2) Palliative surgery to relieve symptoms
      b. Chemotherapy ± radiation = partial response in ≈15%.
      c. Pain control
      d. Control malabsorption
   4. PROGNOSIS
      5-year survival ≈1%.

I. GLOMERULAR SYNDROMES
    A. *Acute nephritic syndrome*
        1. DEFINITION
            a. ↓ renal function
                (1) Fluid retention
                (2) Edema
                (3) ± oliguria
            b. ± hypertension
            c. Nephronal hematuria
                (1) RBC casts
                (2) Dysmorphic RBCs
            d. Proteinuria
                ≈1-3 grams/day
        2. Common etiologies
            a. Postinfectious
                (1) **Poststreptococcal glomerulonephritis**
                (2) Nonstreptococcal postinfectious glomerulonephritis
                    (a) Bacteria
                        ▸ *Streptococcus pneumoniae*
                        ▸ *Staphylococcus* sp.
                        ▸ *Legionella pneumophilia*
                        ▸ Sepsis
                    (b) Virus
                        ▸ Hepatitis B
                        ▸ Varicella
                        ▸ Measles
                        ▸ Mumps
                        ▸ Mononucleosis
                    (c) Spirochete
                      Syphilis
                  (d) Parasites
                      Malaria
            b. Cardiac
                (1) Infective endocarditis
                (2) Venticuloatrial shunts
            c. Multisystem diseases
                (1) Systemic lupus erythematosus
                (2) Henoch-Schönlein purpura
                (3) Vasculitis

B. *Rapidly progressive glomerulonephritis*
    1. DEFINITION
        a. Nephronal hematuria
            (1) RBC casts
            (2) Dysmorphic RBCs
        b. Diffuse glomerular crescent formation
        c. Renal failure developing over weeks to months
    2. Common etiologies
        a. Primary glomerular disease
            (1) Crescentic glomerulonephritis
                (a) Primary
                (b) Idiopathic
            (2) Associated or "superimposed" with another *primary* glomerular disease
                (a) Mesangiocapillary glomerulonephritis
                (b) Membranous glomerulonephritis
        b. Infections
            (1) Poststreptococcal glomerulonephritis
            (2) Infective endocarditis
        c. Multisystem diseases
            (1) Systemic lupus erythematosus
            (2) Henoch-Schönlein purpura
            (3) Vasculitis
C. *Nephrotic syndrome*
    1. DEFINITION
        a. Proteinuria
            >3.5 grams/day
        b. Hypoalbuminemia
        c. Edema
        d. Hyperlipidemia
        e. Lipiduria
    2. ETIOLOGIES
        a. About three quarters are glomerular
            (1) Minimal change disease
            (2) Focal segmental glomerulonephritis
            (3) Membranous glomerulonephritis
            (4) Membranoproliferative glomerulonephritis
        b. About one quarter have a systemic etiology
            (1) Multisystem disease
                (a) Diabetes mellitus
                (b) Systemic lupus erythematosus

   (c) Amyloidosis

   (d) Henoch-Schönlein purpura

  (2) Drugs

   (a) NSAIDs

   (b) Gold

  (3) Infection

   (a) Bacterial

    ▸ Poststreptococcal glomerulonephritis

    ▸ Infective endocarditis

   (b) Viral

    Hepatitis B

  (4) Malignancies

   (a) Lymphomas

   (b) Leukemias

   (c) Cacinomas

II. ACUTE RENAL FAILURE

 A. DEFINITION

  1. Acute ↓ in renal function

   a. *Azotemia*

    ↑ BUN and ↑ creatinine

   b. *Oliguria*

    ↓ Urine output <400 cc/day

   c. *Nonoliguric renal failure*

    A urinary output >400 cc/day

   d. Anuric acute renal failure is uncommon

  2. Three general categories of renal failure

   a. **Prerenal**

    (1) Inadequate perfusion of the kidney

    (2) **The most common cause of *acute* renal failure**

   b. **Intrarenal**

    The pathology is *within* the kidney.

   c. **Postrenal**

    Obstruction of urine flow anywhere from the kidneys to the urethra

  3. Etiologies

   a. *Prerenal failure*

    (1) Cardiovascular

     (a) Congestive heart failure

     (b) Myocardial infarction

     (c) Dysrhythmia

(2) Vascular

(a) Renal artery obstruction

(b) Aortic/renal aneurysm

(3) Hypovolemia

(a) Hemorrhage

(b) Severe vomiting and/or severe diarrhea

(c) Burns

(4) Fluid sequestration

(a) Burns

(b) Shock

▸ Septic

▸ Anaphylaxis

b. *Intrarenal failure*

(1) **Acute Tubular Necrosis**

(a) Responsible for ≈70% of acute renal failure

▸ ≈60% secondary to trauma and surgery

▸ ≈40% secondary to illness

▸ ≈1-2% secondary to pregnancy.

(b) Etiologies

▸ Ischemic

All etiologies of prerenal failure

▸ Nephrotoxic

• Medicinals

∘ Antibiotics and anesthetics

• Heavy metals

• Organic solvents

• Hemolysis

• Rhabdomyolysis

(c) Stages

▸ Stage 1 = Azotemia

▸ Stage 2 = Oliguria

▸ Stage 3 = Diuresis

▸ Stage 4 = Resolving diuresis

(2) Vascular

(a) Vasculitis

(b) Malignant hypertension

(c) Vascular occlusion

(3) Glomerular

Glomerulonephritis

       (4) Interstitial

           Interstitial nephritis

   c. *Postrenal failure*

       (1) Kidneys

           Calculi

       (2) Bladder

          (a) Neoplasm

          (b) Any urethral or bladder neck obstruction

       (3) Prostate

          (a) BPH

          (b) Neoplasm

B. DIAGNOSIS

   1. *Prerenal*

      a. History and physical

         (1) Identify the *underlying* etiology of the hypoperfusion

           (a) Signs and symptoms of

               ▸ Hypovolemia

               ▸ Hypotension

               ▸ Vascular obstruction

               ▸ Fluid sequestration

      b. Laboratory

         (1) CBC, Chem 28, CXR, ECG, will reveal changes diagnostic of underlying pathology.

         (2) Urinalysis

           (a) Few urinary sediments

              ± hyaline casts

   2. *Intrarenal*

      a. History and physical

         (1) *Oliguria* is classic

           Remember 50% of patients with ATN are nonoliguric

         (2) Lethargy

         (3) Fatigue

         (4) Confusion

         (5) Abdominal pain

         (6) Anorexia

         (7) Nausea and vomiting

         (8) Edema

          (a) Periorbital

          (b) Pedal

          (c) Pulmonary

b. Laboratory
    (1) Urinalysis
        (a) ATN
            ‣ Brownish pigmented cellular casts
            ‣ Casts containing renal tubular epithelial cells
        (b) Glomerular lesions
            ‣ Red blood cell casts
            ‣ Proteinuria
            ‣ Red blood cells
        (c) Vascular lesions
            Red blood cell casts
        (d) Interstitial nephritis
            ‣ White cell casts
            ‣ Nonpigmented granular casts

b. Chem-28
    (1) ↑ BUN, ↑ creatinine
    (2) Hyperkalemia
        (a) ECG Changes
            ‣ Bradycardia
            ‣ Peaked T-waves
            ‣ Prolonged QRS and PR interval
    (3) ± hyponatremia
    (4) Hypocalcemia
    (5) Hyperphosphatemia
    (6) Hypermagnesemia
    (7) Hyperuricemia

c. CBC
    (1) Anemia
    (2) ± mild leukocytosis
    (3) ± thrombocytopenia

d. Metabolic acidosis
    ↓ bicarbonate

3. *Postrenal*
    a. History and physical
        (1) Identify the *underlying* etiology of the obstruction
            (a) Abdominal pain
            (b) Flank pain
            (c) ± urine output
                ‣ Dribbling urine
                ‣ Frequency

    (d) Palpable bladder
    (e) Enlarged prostate
    (f) Pelvic masses
  b. Laboratory
   (1) Urinalysis
    (a) ± hyaline casts
    (b) ± crystals
    (c) Leukocytes
    (d) ± hematuria

C. TREATMENT

1. Identify and treat all prerenal and postrenal pathology as quickly as possible
2. Identify and treat any intrarenal pathology as quickly as possible
3. Establish urinary output
 Fluids and/or diuretics
4. **Conservative medical management**
 a. Monitor fluid status
  (1) Correct any intravacular fluid depletion
  (2) Correct any intravascular fluid overload
   (a) Intake and output
     500 ccs + the number of cc's output in the previous 24 hours
  (3) Daily weights
 b. Modify diet
  (1) Restrict dietary protein
   (a) 0.5 g/kg of body weight/day
   (b) ↑ essential amino acids
  (2) Carbohydrates for calories
 c. Serial monitoring of electrolytes/kidney function
  (1) BUN and Creatinine
  (2) Electrolytes
   (a) **Correct hyperkalemia**
   (b) **Correct hyperphosphatemia**
   (c) Correct hypocalcemia
   (d) Correct hyponatremia
   (e) Correct hyperuricemia
  (3) Avoid magnesium-containing compounds
 d. **Correct the metabolic acidosis**
 e. Adjust medication dosages
 f. Treat any underlying infections
 g. Correct any anemia
 h. **Dialysis does not appear to hasten recovery in acute renal failure**

5. Indications for Dialysis
 a. Progressive azotemia
  (1) BUN >100
  (2) Creatinine >10 mEq/dL
 b. Severe metabolic acidosis
  Serum bicarbonate <10 mEq/L following therapy
 c. Severe hyperkalemia
  Serum potassium >6.5 mEq/L
 d. Pulmonary edema secondary to fluid overload
 e. Neurologic deterioration
  (1) Seizures
  (2) Encephalopathy
 f. GI bleeding
 g. Pericarditis

D. PROGNOSIS
 1. The mortality rate is dependent upon the etiology of acute renal failure
  a. Trauma including burns and major surgery... ≈60%
  b. Toxin-related.. ≈30%
  c. Obstetrical patients.................................... ≈15%
 2. Overall, the mortality rate is................................. ≈50%

III. **CHRONIC RENAL FAILURE**
 A. DEFINITION
  1. Chronic renal failure
   The *permanent* loss of renal function
  2. **Uremia**
   The constellation of signs and symptoms of advanced renal failure
  3. Etiologies
   a. *Diabetes Mellitus*............................≈30%
   b. *Hypertension*..................................≈25%
   c. *Glomerulonephritis*.........................≈15%
   d. Cystic renal disease.........................≈ 4%
   e. Miscellaneous Urologic disease.........≈ 6%
   f. Other systemic illness.......................≈ 6%
   g. Unknown......................................≈14%
 B. DIAGNOSIS
  1. History and physical
   a. Skin
    (1) Ecchymosis
    (2) Pruritus

(3) Uremic frost
b. Cardiovascular
(1) Hypertension
(2) Pericarditis
(3) CHF
c. Neurologic
(1) Fatigue
(2) Peripheral neuropathy
(3) Encephalopathy
(4) Confusion
d. Musculoskeletal
(1) Muscle pain
(2) Osteomalacia
(3) Osteoporosis
e. Gastrointestinal
(1) Anorexia
(2) Nausea and vomiting
(3) Peptic ulcer disease
(4) Gastroenteritis
f. Hematologic
(1) Hemorrhage
(2) Anemia
g. Pulmonary
(1) Pneumonia
(2) Pulmonary edema
(3) Uremic lung
2. Laboratory
a. CBC
(1) Normochromic, normocytic anemia
(2) ↓ red blood cell mass
(3) Lymphopenia
(4) ± leukopenia
(5) Thrombocytopenia
b. Chem-28
(1) ↑ BUN
(2) ↑ creatinine
(3) ↓ sodium levels
(4) Hyperkalemia only in the final stages of renal failure
(5) Hypocalcemia
(6) Hyperphosphatemia

(7) Hyperuricemia

(8) Hypermagnesemia

c. Metabolic acidosis

d. Urinalysis

(1) Proteinuria

(2) Urine sediment dependent upon underlying pathology

C. TREATMENT

1. Try to maintain urine output for as long as possible

Balance between fluids and/or diuretics

2. **Conservative medical management**

a. Monitor fluid status

b. Modified diet

c. Monitoring of electrolytes/kidney function

d. Correct the metabolic acidosis

e. Adjust medication dosages

f. Treat any underlying infections

g. Treat the anemia

(1) Erythropoietin

(2) Transfusion

h. Treat any hypertension

3. **Indications for Dialysis**

a. Progressive azotemia

(1) BUN >100

(2) Creatinine >10 mEq/dL

b. Severe metabolic acidosis

Serum bicarbonate <10 mEq/L following therapy

c. Severe hyperkalemia

Serum potassium >6.5 mEq/L

d. Pulmonary edema secondary to fluid overload

e. Neurologic deterioration

(1) Seizures

(2) Encephalopathy

f. GI bleeding

g. Pericarditis

4. Transplantation

I. KIDNEY
  A. *Acute Pyelonephritis*
    1. DEFINITION
       a. An infection of the collecting system and/or renal parenchyma usually caused by a bacteria.
       b. Bacteremia and sepsis can occur.
       c. Etiologies (Most common)
          (1) Enterobacteriaceae
              (a) *Escherichia coli*
              (b) *Proteus* sp.
              (c) *Klebsiella* sp.
              (d) *Enterobacter* sp.
              (e) *Pseudomonas* sp.
          (2) Enterococcus
          (3) *Staphylococcus saprophyticus*
          (4) *Staphylococcus aureus*
    2. DIAGNOSIS
       a. History and physical
          (1) Back pain or CVA tenderness
          (2) Fever
          (3) ± chills
          (4) Nausea and vomiting
          (5) Diarrhea
       b. Laboratory
          (1) Urinalysis
              (a) Leukocytes
              (b) **White blood cell casts**
              (c) ± hematuria
              (d) Sediment
                  ‣ Gram stain + for bacteria
                  ‣ **Pyuria = >10 WBCs/HPF**
          (2) Urine culture and sensitivity
          (3) CBC
                  Leukocytosis
          (4) Blood cultures in severe illness
    3. TREATMENT
       a. A 14-day course of therapy is usually sufficient
       b. **Avoid amoxicillin or ampicillin since 20-30% of *E coli* are resistant**
       c. Mild to moderate infection
          (1) Trimethoprim-Sulfamethoxazole
          (2) Fluoroquinolones

   d. Severe disease
    (1) Hospitalization
    (2) IV quinolones or
    (3) Aminoglycoside and/or third generation cephalosporin
    (4) Watch for signs and symptoms of sepsis
    (5) Supportive care as needed
    (6) Following identification of bacteria and response to IV meds, change to oral medication.
   e. Pregnancy
    (1) Hospitalization
    (2) IV cephalosporin or extended-spectrum penicillin
  4. COMPLICATIONS
   a. Renal abscess
   b. Perinephric abscess
   c. Sepsis
B. *Nephrolithiasis*
  1. DEFINITION
   a. The formation of calculi (stones) within the kidney
   b. A calculi
    (1) Crystalline substance + an organic matrix.
     (a) **Calcium stones**..............≈**75%**
     (b) Struvite stones...............≈15%
     (c) Uric acid stones.............≈ 8%
     (d) Cystine stones................≈ 2%
   c. **Calculi can cause obstruction and infection**.
   d. Etiologies
    (1) Calcium stones
     (a) Hypercalciuria
      Urine calcium excretion >4 mg/kg/24 hours
     (b) Idiopathic nephrolithiasis
      ▸ Hypercalciuria + normal serum calcium
      ▸ Causes the majority of stone formation
      ▸ Two mechanisms
       • "Renal" hypercalciuria
        ↑ calcium absorption in the intestine *secondary* to a defect in renal calcium reabsorption in the kidney.
       • "Absorptive" hypercalciuria
        ↑ intestinal absorption drives ↑ calcium excretion

        (c) Secondary hypercalciuria
- Hypercalciuria + hypercalcemia
- Hyperparathyroidism
- Sarcoidosis
- Hypervitaminosis D
- Primary or metastatic neoplasm to the bone
- Distal renal tubular acidosis

     (2) Struvite stones

        (a) "Infection stone"

        (b) An abnormally alkaline urine secondary to the formation of ammonia from urea, by urea-splitting bacteria, form $MgNH_4PO_4$
- Urea splitting bacteria
  - *Proteus* sp.
  - *Pseudomonas* sp.

     (3) Uric acid stones

        (a) ↑ urinary uric acid

        (b) Chronic acidity of urine

        (c) Chronic dehydration

     (4) Cystine stones

        (a) Genetic disorder

           Cystinuria an autosomal recessive inherited disorder

2. DIAGNOSIS

  a. History and physical

     (1) **"Renal colic"**

        (a) Severe flank pain

        (b) Radiation of the pain to the groin

     (2) **Microscopic hematuria**

     (3) **Nausea ± vomiting**

     (4) Tachycardia

     (5) Diaphoresis

     (6) Frequency

     (7) Dysuria

  b. Laboratory

     (1) Urinalysis

        (a) **Hematuria**

        (b) ± pyuria

        (c) Urine sediment

           + for crystals

     (2) CBC

        ± leukocytosis

(3) Chem 28
    (a) Check BUN and creatinine
    (b) Check the calcium, phosphorus, uric acid
(4) Urine cultures
(5) Plain film of the abdomen
    ≈90% of kidney stones are radiopaque.
(6) IVP
    (a) Identifies radiolucent stones
    (b) Identifies location and extent of obstruction.

3. TREATMENT
    a. ↑ fluids
    b. Pain medication
    c. Strain urine for stone
    d. **Stone analysis**
    e. Dependent upon stone analysis
        (1) ↑ **fluids**
        (2) Modify diet
        (3) **Treat the *underlying* disease**
            (a) Calcium
                ▸ ± thiazide diuretic
                ▸ ± neutral phosphate
                ▸ ± cellulose phosphate
                ▸ ± magnesium oxide
            (b) Struvite
                ▸ Remove the stone
                ▸ Treat the infection
            (c) Uric acid
                ▸ Treat hyperuricosuria with allopurinol
                ▸ Alkalinization of the urine
    f. Most stones <4 mm pass spontaneously
    g. If a stone doesn't pass
        (1) Endo-urologic stone removal
        (2) Lithotripsy
        (3) Surgery

C. NEOPLASM
    1. *Renal cell carcinoma*
        a. DEFINITION
            (1) A primary *adenocarcinoma* of the kidney probably arising from the proximal tubular cells.

(2) It is an unpredictable tumor with variable growth patterns.

(3) 85% of all primary renal tumors

b. DIAGNOSIS

    (1) History and physical

        (a) The *classic triad* of gross hematuria, flank pain and flank mass occurs ≈10% of the time

        (b) **Painless hematuria**

        (c) Flank pain

        (d) Flank mass

        (e) Weight loss

        (f) Fever

        (g) Fatigue

        (h) Anorexia

    (2) Laboratory

        (a) CBC

            Anemia

        (b) Urinalysis

           ▸ Hematuria

           ▸ Proteinuria

           ▸ ± neoplastic cells in sediment

        (c) ↑ ESR

        (d) Hyperglobulinemia

        (e) **IVP**

            Intravenous pyelography detects most renal masses

        (f) Ultrasonography delineates cystic and solid lesions

        (g) **CT or MRI of kidney**

            Defines the lesion and helps determine direct extension or abdominal metastasis.

c. TREATMENT

    (1) Surgery is the treatment of choice

    (2) Radiation therapy

        (a) No role in early disease

        (b) Palliate symptoms of metastatic bone and CNS lesions

    (3) Chemotherapy

        No role in early disease

d. PROGNOSIS

    (1) Five-year survival

        (a) Stage I................≈50-60%

        (b) Stage IV...................<5%

2. *Wilms' tumor (Nephroblastoma)*

    a. DEFINITION

        (1) A malignant renal tumor composed of mixed embryonal cell elements.

        (2) A childhood tumor in which familial clusters have been described.

        (3) ↑ mature elements + ↓ anaplastic cells = best prognosis.

    b. DIAGNOSIS

        (1) History and physical

            (a) Painless hematuria

            (b) Abdominal pain

            (c) Enlarged abdomen

            (d) ± palpable abdominal mass

        (2) Laboratory

            (a) CT or MRI of abdomen is diagnostic for mass

            (b) Urinalysis

                Hematuria

    c. TREATMENT

        (1) Surgery

            Nephrectomy

        (2) Radiation therapy

        (3) Chemotherapy

    d. PROGNOSIS

        (1) Two-year survival

            (a) Stage I, II, and III.........≈95%

            (b) Stage IV......................≈50%

II. BLADDER

    A. *Cystitis*

        1. DEFINITION

            a. An infection of the bladder

            b. Etiologies

                 (1) Enterobacteriaceae

                     (a) *E coli*

                     (b) *Proteus* sp.

                     (c) *Klebsiella sp.*

                     (d) *Enterobacter* sp.

                     (e) *Pseudomonas* sp.

                 (2) Enterococcus

                 (3) ***Staphylococcus saprophyticus***

                     The second most common pathogen in women

                 (4) *Staphylococcus aureus*

2. DIAGNOSIS
    a. History and Physical
        (1) Suprapubic tenderness
        (2) Frequency
        (3) Dysuria
        (4) Urgency
    b. Laboratory
        (1) Urinalysis
            (a) Leukocytes
            (b) ± hematuria
            (c) Sediment
                ▸ Gram stain + for bacteria
                ▸ Pyuria = >10 WBCs/HPF
        (2) Urine culture and sensitivity
3. TREATMENT
    a. **Avoid amoxicillin or ampicillin since 20-40% of *E coli* are resistant**
    b. Trimethoprim-Sulfamethoxazole
    c. Quinolones
    d. Cephalosporins
    e. Nitrofurantoin
    f. Treat for 10-14 days.

B. *Bladder Cancer*
  1. DEFINITION
    a. A primary malignancy of the bladder
    b. ↑ risk factors
        (1) Aniline dye workers
        (2) Exposure to chemicals in paint, rubber and leather industry
        (3) Smoking
    c. Histologic classification
        (1) **Transitional cell (Urothelial) ≈90%.**
            Less aggressive
        (2) Squamous cell ≈8%
            More aggressive
  2. DIAGNOSIS
    a. History and Physical
        (1) **Hematuria**
        (2) Dysuria
        (3) Frequency
        (4) Suprapubic tenderness
        (5) Postvoiding pain

        (6) Urgency

        (7) Hesitancy

    b. Laboratory

        (1) **Cystoscopy with transurethral biopsy**

            The procedure of choice in diagnosing bladder cancer

3. TREATMENT

    a. Superficial lesions ≈85% of all bladder cancers

    b. ↑ the depth of invasion the more radical the therapy

    c. Surgery

        (1) Early disease

            Transurethral resection + intravesical chemotherapy

        (2) Patients must be followed closely for recurrence.

        (3) Late disease

            Radical cystectomy with lymph node dissection

    d. Radiation therapy is not indicated

    e. Chemotherapy

        (1) Intravesical for early disease

        (2) Combination therapy for advanced disease

4. PROGNOSIS

    a. 5-year survival

        (1) Stage 0 Papillary mucosal lesion..............≈80%

        (2) Stage D Metastases in draining nodes......<10%

    b. ↑ the depth of invasion the worse the prognosis

III. URETHRA

    A. *Urethritis*

        1. DEFINITION

            a. An infection of the urethra characterized by dysuria and discharge.

            b. The urethritis may be gonococcal or nongonococcal in origin

            c. Etiology of gonococcal urethritis

                Neisseria gonorrhoeae

            d. Etiologies of nongonococcal urethritis

                (1) *Chlamydia trachomatis*..**30-50%**

                (2) *Ureaplasma urealyticum*...20-25%

                (3) *Trichomonas vaginalis*, *Herpes simplex* and *Candida*........1-5%

                (4) Unknown etiology..20-30%

            e. ≈ 10% of nongonococcal urethritis is asymptomatic

            f. **Gonococcal and chlamydial infection present a different clinical syndrome in women.**

2. DIAGNOSIS
   a. History and Physical
      (1) **Urethral discharge**
         (a) Gonococcal

         Abrupt onset of a greenish-yellow discharge 1-7 days following exposure
         (b) Nongonococcal

         Gradual onset of a clear to mucoid white discharge 10-14 days following exposure
      (2) Dysuria
      (3) Meatal itching, erythema, tenderness
      (4) ± suprapubic tenderness
   b. Laboratory
      (1) Gonorrhea
         (a) Gram stain of discharge

         Gram-negative intracellular diplococci *within* neutrophils.
         (b) Immunodiagnostic antigen detection of gonococcus from discharge
         (c) Confirm with culture
      (2) Chlamydia
         (a) Gram stain of discharge

         Neutrophils only
         (b) Confirm with negative gonorrhea culture
         (c) Immunodiagnostic antigen detection of chlamydia from discharge

3. TREATMENT
   a. Uncomplicated gonococcal urethritis
      (1) Ceftriaxone 125-250 mg IM or
      (2) Cifixime 400 mg orally as a single dose or
      (3) Ciprofloxacin 500 mg or Ofloxacin 400 mg orally as a single dose or
      (4) Spectinomycin 2 g. IM
      (5) **All of the above should be followed with doxycycline 100 mg PO bid for 7 days or azithromycin 1 gram orally in a single dose.**
      (6) Pregnant or allergic patients should be placed on Erythromycin 500 mg PO qid x 7 days.
      (7) **Evaluate and treat sexual partners.**
      (8) Test of cure following completion of therapy
   b. Nongonococcal urethritis
      (1) Doxycycline 100 mg PO bid x 7 days or
      (2) Erythromycin 500 mg PO qid x 7 days or
      (3) Azithromycin 1 gram orally in a single dose or
      (4) Ofloxacin 300 mg PO bid x 7 days

(5) **Evaluate and treat sexual partners.**

(6) Test of cure following completion of therapy

IV. **PROSTATE**

    A. *Prostatitis*

        1. DEFINITION

            a. An infection *or* inflammation of the prostate gland

            b. *Acute Bacterial Prostatitis*

                (1) Etiologies

                    (a) Enterobacteriaceae

                    (b) *Pseudomonas* sp.

                (2) An acute infection of the prostate characterized by the rapid onset of:

                    (a) Fever

                    (b) Chills

                    (c) Pain

                          ‣ Perineal

                          ‣ Low back

                          ‣ Suprapubic

                    (d) A hot "boggy" tender gland

                    (e) Dysuria

                    (f) Frequency

                    (g) Urgency

                    (h) ± urinary obstruction

                (3) Laboratory

                    (a) Urinalysis

                          ‣ Pyuria

                          ‣ Bacteriuria

                          ‣ ± macrophages laden with fat droplets

                    (b) CBC

                    Leukocytosis

            c. *Chronic Prostatitis*

                (1) Implicated as a common cause of *recurrent* urinary tract infections

                (2) Signs and symptoms

                    (a) Symptoms may be absent

                    (b) Dysuria

                    (c) Frequency

                    (d) Pain

                        ‣ Suprapubic

                        ‣ Perineal

                        ‣ On ejaculation

(3) Laboratory

    (a) Expressed prostatic secretions

        ▸ >10 cells/HPF

        ▸ >2 lipid laden macrophages/HPF.

        ▸ + culture

d. *Nonbacterial prostatitis*

    (1) Signs and symptoms are similar to chronic prostatitis

    (2) Expressed prostatic secretions >10 cells/HPF but all cultures are negative.

e. *Prostatodynia*

    (1) Signs and symptoms are similar to chronic prostatitis

    (2) Expressed prostatic secretions are normal and all cultures are negative.

3. TREATMENT

    a. Acute bacterial prostatitis

        (1) Hospitalization if acutely ill.

            (a) IV meds

                ▸ Ciprofloxacin or ofloxacin or

                ▸ Aminoglycoside + Ampicillin

        (2) After initial response and identification of organism change to oral meds

            (a) Trimethoprim-Sulfamethoxazole

            (b) Ciprofloxacin

        (3) Catheterize if there is urinary retention

        (4) Fluids

        (5) Pain meds

        (6) Treat 4-6 weeks

        (7) Recheck the expressed prostatic secretions at twelve weeks

    b. Chronic bacterial prostatitis

        (1) Trimethoprim-Sulfamethoxazole

        (2) Ciprofloxacin

        (3) Treat for 4-12 weeks

    c. Nonbacterial prostatitis and prostatodynia

        (1) ± antibiotics depending on signs and symptoms

            Doxycycline

        (2) "Stress management" with associated ↓ in stress improves or cures the condition in a high percentage of cases.

        (3) Terazosin for external urinary sphincter

B. *Benign Prostatic Hypertrophy*

    1. DEFINITION

        a. A *benign* condition characterized by adenomatous, stromal or muscular hyperplasia of the prostate.

b. BPH is rare before 40 years and clinically begins to present after age 50.

c. ↑ size of the prostate compresses the urethra causing obstruction.

2. DIAGNOSIS

a. History and Physical

(1) ↓ force of urine stream

(2) Hesitancy

(3) Frequency

(4) Urgency

(5) Nocturia

(6) Incomplete emptying

(7) Urinary retention

(8) ↑ size of the prostate on digital exam

b. Laboratory

(1) Urinalysis

Check for infection, hematuria

(2) ↑ post-voiding residual urine

(3) BUN and creatinine

Check for postrenal azotemia

(4) PSA

To help rule out underlying malignancy

(5) Ultrasound

(a) Prostatic size

(b) Residual urine volume

(6) Cystourethroscopy

Evaluate urethra, bladder neck and bladder for *other* diseases that cause obstruction.

(7) Intravenous pyelogram

Part of the evaluation if hematuria is present.

(8) Urodynamics

Used to help differentiate the neurological basis of obstructive symptoms

3. TREATMENT

a. General

(1) Avoid caffeine and alcohol

(2) Avoid OTC sympathomimetics

(3) Avoid OTC anticholinergics

b. Medical

(1) Alpha blockade

(a) Terazosin

(b) Prazosin

     (2) 5-alpha-reductase inhibitor
      Finasteride
   c. Surgical
     (1) TUIP (Transurethral incision of the prostate)
     (2) TUDP (Transurethral dilation of prostatic urethra)
     (3) TURP (Transurethral resection of the prostate)
     (4) Transurethral laser ablation
     (5) Open prostatectomy
C. *Prostatic Cancer*
 1. DEFINITION
   a. A primary malignancy of the prostate.
   b. >95% are *adenocarcinoma*.
   c. Many times the cancer is multifocal and may involve the gland's capsule
 2. DIAGNOSIS
   a. History and Physical
     (1) Early disease is asymptomatic
     (2) Advanced disease
       (a) Hesitancy
       (b) Urgency
       (c) ↓ urine stream
       (d) ± hematuria
     (3) Induration or nodularity on digital exam
      Nodules are hard and *not* tender
   b. Laboratory
     (1) **PSA**
       (a) A specific marker for prostate cancer
       (b) Obtain *before* digital exam
     (2) **Needle biopsy**
      Usual method of diagnosis
 3. TREATMENT
   a. Early disease
     (1) Surgery and/or
      Radical prostatectomy
     (2) Radiation therapy
     (3) Chemotherapy or hormone therapy is not indicated
   b. Advanced disease
     (1) Surgery
      TURP to relieve obstruction
     (2) Radiation therapy

(3) Endocrine therapy
    (a) DES
    (b) LHRH agonists
    (c) Orchiectomy
(4) Chemotherapy

4. PROGNOSIS
  a. Ten-year survival
    (1) Stage A
      A single area of well differentiated tumor......................≈60%
    (2) Advanced disease...≈10-20%

V. TESTICLE

  A. *Epididymitis*
    1. DEFINITION
      a. An inflammation of the epididymis that is usually unilateral
      b. Etiologies
        (1) Idiopathic
          ≈50% of the time
        (2) Gram-negative enteric bacilli
    2. DIAGNOSIS
      a. History and Physical
        (1) Scrotal pain
        (2) Enlarged indurated epididymis
        (3) ± fever and chills
        (4) ± urethral discharge
      b. Laboratory
        (1) Urinalysis
          (a) Leukocytes
          (b) ± hematuria
        (2) CBC
          ± leukocytosis
        (3) Gram stain of urethral discharge
        (4) Ultrasound to rule out torsion
    3. TREATMENT
      a. Scrotal support and elevation
      b. Ice
      c. Pain meds
      d. Antibiotics
        (1) <35 years of age
          Doxycycline 100 mg bid x 10 days

(2) >35 years of age
    (a) Trimethoprim-sulfamethoxazole
    (b) Ciprofloxacin
(3) Treat for 7-10 days

B. *Testicular Cancer*
  1. DEFINITION
    a. A primary malignancy of the testicle.
    b. Histologic typing of tumors
      (1) Seminomas.........................≈40-50%
      (2) Embryonal cell/teratoma..........≈50%
      (3) Choriocarcinoma.....................< 1%
    c. **Cryptorchid testicle ↑ risk of seminoma by 10-40%**
  2. DIAGNOSIS
    a. History and Physical
      (1) Testicular enlargement ± pain.
      (2) ± lymphadenopathy
        (a) Inguinal
        (b) Iliac
        (c) Supraclavicular nodes
    b. Laboratory
      (1) Tumor markers
        (a) ∝-Fetoprotein
        (b) β-hCG
      (2) CT of chest
        ↑ detection of metastatic disease
      (3) CT of abdomen
        Evaluation of retroperitoneal disease
  3. TREATMENT
    a. Seminoma (Stage A and B)
      (1) Surgery
        Transinguinal orchiectomy
      (2) Radiation therapy
        Retroperitoneal nodes
      (3) **Seminomas are ↑ sensitive to radiation**
    b. Seminoma (Stage C)
      Chemotherapy

      c. Nonseminomatous germ cell cancers (Stage A and B)

          (1) Surgery

               Transinguinal orchiectomy and retroperitoneal lymph node dissection

          (2) Radiation therapy is not indicated in early disease.

          (3) Chemotherapy is highly effective

4. PROGNOSIS

      a. 5-year survival for seminoma

          Stage A.......................... ≈95-99%

      b. 5-year survival for nonseminomatous tumor

          Stage C............................. ≈70%

I. VULVA/VAGINA

A. Vulvar and Vaginal Infections

    1. *Candida Vulvovaginitis*

        a. DEFINITION

            An inflammation of the vulva and/or vagina by *Candida albicans* or non-albicans yeast forms.

        b. DIAGNOSIS

            (1) History and Physical

                (a) **Vulvar and/or vaginal itching and/or burning**

                (b) Vulvar erythema

                (c) White, "cottage cheese" discharge

                (d) Odorless

            (2) Laboratory

                (a) A normal vaginal pH (≤ 4.5)

                (b) Wet preps

                    Branched and budding pseudohyphae.

        c. TREATMENT

            (1) Miconazole, clotrimazole or terconazole cream or suppositories.

            (2) Oral fluconazole or ketoconazole

    2. *Trichomonal vaginitis*

        a. DEFINITION

            An inflammation of the vagina caused by the protozoan *Trichomonas vaginalis.*

        b. DIAGNOSIS

            (1) History and Physical

                (a) A thin watery yellowish-green to greenish-grey discharge

                (b) Frothy, foul smelling discharge

                (c) ± dysuria

                (d) Vulvar and vaginal erythema/edema

                (e) Vaginal itching and burning

            (2) Laboratory

                (a) Vaginal pH = 5-5.5

                (b) Wet preps

                    + for trichomonads

        c. TREATMENT

            (1) Metronidazole

                (a) 2 grams in a single oral dose has a cure rate $\approx 90\%$.

                (b) Failure of therapy or severe infection

                    Metronidazole 250 mg three times a day for a week.

(2) **Treat the patient and the partner.**

(3) **Avoid ETOH because of "antabuse" effect.**

(4) Do not use metronidazole in the first trimester of pregnancy.

3. *Gardnerella vaginitis*

    a. DEFINITION

        A vaginal infection caused by the bacteria *Gardnerella vaginalis*.

    b. DIAGNOSIS

        (1) History and Physical

            A greyish-white discharge with a characteristic foul or fishy odor.

        (2) Laboratory

            (a) Vaginal pH >5.0

            (b) Wet Preps

                ▸ **Clue cells**

                    Epithelial cells with bacilli clinging to their surface

    c. TREATMENT

        (1) Clindamycin cream

        (2) Metronidazole 250-500 mg. three times a day for a week

        (3) **Treat the patient and partner.**

        (4) **Avoid ETOH because of "Antabuse" effect.**

II. CERVIX

    A. *Cervicitis*

        1. DEFINITION

            a. An acute or chronic inflammation of the endocervix

            b. Etiologies of *acute cervicitis*

                (1) Infection

                    (a) *Neisseria gonorrhoeae*

                    (b) *Trichomonas vaginalis*

                    (c) *Herpes Simplex*

                    (d) *Chlamydia trachomatis*

                (2) Trauma

                (3) Malignancy

                (4) Radiation therapy

             c. Etiology of *chronic cervicitis*

                (1) Idiopathic

                (2) Postmenopausal

        2. DIAGNOSIS

            a. History and Physical

                (1) Vaginal discharge

                (2) Postcoital spotting and/or bleeding

(3) Dyspareunia

(4) Erythema of cervix

(5) Friable cervix which bleeds easily upon examination

(6) ± mucopurulent discharge from the cervical os

(7) ± cervical ulcerations

b. Laboratory

(1) Endocervical Gram stain >10 WBCs/HPF is suggestive of cervicitis

(2) *Neisseria gonorrhoeae*

(a) Gram stain

▸ + for gram-negative intracellular diplococci

▸ **Beware, in women, false + secondary to saprophytic *Neisseria* spp.**

(b) Confirm with culture

(3) *Trichomonas vaginalis*

(a) + wet prep

(b) + Gram stain

(c) + pap smear

(4) *Herpes Simplex*

(a) + culture

(b) + cellular changes on pap smear

(c) + herpes virus antibody titers

(5) *Chlamydia trachomatis*

(a) + culture

(b) + cellular changes on pap smear

3. TREATMENT

a. Cervicitis secondary to suspected gonococcal or chlamydial infection should be treated while cultures are pending

Ceftriaxone 125-250 mg IM *followed by* **doxycycline 100 mg BID x 7 days**

b. *Herpes Simplex*

Acyclovir

c. Trichomonas

Metronidazole

d. Chronic cervicitis

(1) Estrogen creams for postmenopausal cervical inflammation.

(2) Sulfonamide vaginal creams

B. *Cervical Dysplasia*

1. DEFINITION

A disorder characterized by abnormal squamous cell cytology which reflect neoplastic epithelial changes in the transformation zone of the cervix.

2. DIAGNOSIS
    a. History and Physical
        (1) **The patient may be asymptomatic**
        (2) ± vaginal discharge
        (3) ± postcoital spotting or bleeding
    b. Laboratory
        (1) Pap Smear
            (a) Class system
                ▸ Class I...........Normal
                ▸ Class II..........Inflammatory Atypia
                ▸ Class III.......Dysplasia
                ▸ Class IV.......Carcinoma in situ
                ▸ Class V..........Invasive carcinoma
            (b) Cervical intraepithelial classification
                ▸ CIN I.............Mild to moderate dysplasia
                ▸ CIN II...........Moderate to severe dysplasia
                ▸ CIN III..........Carcinoma in situ

3. TREATMENT
    a. Class I pap smear
        Yearly pap smear
    b. Class II pap smear
        (1) Treat the underlying inflammation
        (2) Recheck in 4-6 months until three negative smears have been reported and
            then return to yearly screening
        (3) If atypia is persistent follow protocol for class III or greater pap smear
    c. Class III, IV, V pap smear
        (1) Colposcopy with directed biopsy and endocervical curettage
        (2) If CIN I (mild to moderate dysplasia) with negative endocervical curettage
            (a) Cryocautery
            (b) Laser therapy
        (3) **Repeat pap smear in three month**
            (a) If normal, repeat in six months and if normal yearly follow-up
            (b) If abnormal, reevaluation and retreatment
        (4) If CIN II or III (Severe dysplasia or carcinoma in situ) or + endocervical
            curettage
            (a) Therapeutic cone
                ▸ **Repeat pap smear in three month**
                    • If normal, repeat in six months and if normal yearly
                      follow-up
                    • If abnormal, reevaluation and retreatment

            (b) Consider hysterectomy *if* childbearing isn't a factor

        (5) Invasive cancer

            (a) Surgery

            (b) Radiation

C. *Cervical Cancer*

    1. DEFINITION

        a. A primary malignancy of the uterine cervix

        b. ↑ risk of cervical cancer

            (1) Early, frequent intercourse

            (2) Multiple sexual partners

            (3) Early first pregnancy

            (4) High parity

            (5) HPV infection

            (6) Smoking

        c. Histology

            (1) **Squamous cell carcinomas...≈80% of cases**

            (2) Adenocarcinomas..................≈18% of cases

    2. DIAGNOSIS

        a. History and Physical

            (1) **The patient may be asymptomatic**

            (2) Vaginal discharge may be present

            (3) Postcoital spotting or bleeding

            (4) ± cervical mass noted on pelvic exam

        b. Laboratory

            (1) Pap smear

            (2) Biopsy

        c. Staging

            (1) Stage 0......Carcinoma in situ

            (2) Stage I...... Confined to the cervix

            (3) Stage II.....Beyond cervix but *not* involving pelvic wall or upper third of the vagina.

            (4) Stage III....Extension to the pelvic wall *or* lower third of the vagina.

            (5) Stage IV....Distant metastases or involvement of bladder or rectal mucosa.

    3. TREATMENT

            (1) Stage 0

                (a) Therapeutic cone

                    ▸ **Repeat pap smear in three month**

                        • If normal, repeat in six months and if normal yearly follow-up

                        • If abnormal, reevaluation and retreatment

(b) Consider hysterectomy *if* childbearing isn't a factor
(2) Stages Ia1 and Ia2
    (a) Lesions <7 mm in diameter, no lymph-vascular space invasion and *<3 mm of stromal invasion*
        ▸ Excisional conization
        ▸ Consider hysterectomy *if* childbearing isn't a factor
    (b) Lesions <7 mm in diameter, no lymph-vascular space invasion and *3-5 mm of stromal invasion*
        Radical hysterectomy with bilateral pelvic lymphadenectomy
(3) Stages Ib and IIa
    (a) Radical hysterectomy with bilateral pelvic lymphadenectomy and para-aortic lymph node evaluation
    (b) Poor surgical candidates
        Radiation therapy
(4) Stages IIb and III
    (a) Radiation therapy
    (b) Chemotherapy
(5) Stage IV
    (a) Radiation therapy
    (b) Pelvic exenteration
    (c) Chemotherapy

4. PROGNOSIS
    a. Five-year survival
        (1) Stage 0..............≈95-100%
        (2) Stage I....................≈80%
        (3) Stage II...................≈60%
        (4) Stage III.................≈30%
        (5) Stage IV...................≈5%

III. UTERUS
    A. NEOPLASIA
        1. *Leiomyoma*
            a. DEFINITION
                (1) A uterine leiomyomata is a *benign* smooth muscle tumor
                (2) It is also called a fibroid tumor
                (3) Classification by location
                    (a) Submucous
                    (b) Intramural
                    (c) Subserosal

(4) They are highly estrogen dependent.
b. DIAGNOSIS
    (1) History and Physical
        (a) Most are asymptomatic
        (b) Menorrhagia
        (c) Pelvic pressure or "heaviness"
        (d) Pelvic pain
        (e) Frequency and urgency of urination
        (f) Dyspareunia
        (g) Dysmenorrhea
        (h) ↑ tumors are palpable
    (2) Laboratory
        Pelvic ultrasound can readily identify this lesion.
c. TREATMENT
    (1) Observation
    (2) Myomectomy to ↓ problems during intended pregnancy.
    (3) Surgery
        (a) When the uterus reaches 12-14 week size or
        (b) Abnormal uterine bleeding or
        (c) Severe pain

2. *Endometrial carcinoma*
    a. DEFINITION
        (1) A primary malignancy of the endometrium of the uterus.
        (2) Postmenopausal women..................≈80% of cases
        (3) Histology
            (a) Adenocarcinomas................≈70% of cases
            (b) Adenocanthomas....................≈20% of cases
            (c) Adenosquamous carcinoma....≈10% of cases
    b. DIAGNOSIS
        (1) History and Physical
            (a) Abnormal vaginal bleeding
                ▸ Premenopausal
                    • Hypermenorrhea
                    • Menorrhagia
                    • Metrorrhagia
                    • Menometrorrhagia
                ▸ Postmenopausal
                  Vaginal bleeding one year following cessation of
                  menstrual cycle

(2) Laboratory

    (a) Endocervical curettage

    (b) Endometrial biopsy

    (c) Fractional curettage of the uterus is the diagnostic test of choice

(3) Staging

    (a) Stage O.....Carcinoma in situ

    (b) Stage I......Confined to the corpus

    (c) Stage II.....Corpus + cervix but *not* extending outside of the uterus

    (d) Stage III....Extends outside the uterus but *not* the true pelvis

    (e) Stage IV....Extends outside the pelvis *or* invades the bladder or rectal mucosa.

c. TREATMENT

(1) Stages I and II

    (a) Total hysterectomy with bilateral salpingo-oophorectomy

    (b) ± lymphadenectomy

    (c) Radiation therapy

        ▸ For high-risk surgical patients

        ▸ Pre-op for high-grade cancers

        ▸ Post-op for metastatic lymph node disease or for high-grade tumors

    (d) Chemotherapy has no role in early disease

(2) Stages III and IV

    (a) Total hysterectomy with bilateral salpingo-oophorectomy

    (b) Surgical removal of macroscopic disease

    (c) Radiation therapy

        ▸ External beam therapy

        ▸ Implantation

    (d) Hormone therapy

        ▸ Progesterone

        ▸ Tamoxifen

    (e) Chemotherapy

d. PROGNOSIS

(1) Five-year survival

    (a) Stage I......................≈85%

    (b) Stage II....................≈60%

    (c) Stage III..................≈35%

    (d) Stage IV..................≈10%

IV. FALLOPIAN TUBES
   A. *Ectopic pregnancy*
   1. DEFINITION
      a. Implantation of the fertilized ovum *outside* the endometrial cavity.
      b. Location
         Fallopian tube ≈95% of the time
      c. Etiology
         Although intrinsic abnormalities of fertilized ovum occur, damage to the endosalpinx secondary to sexually transmitted disease plays a significant role.
   2. DIAGNOSIS
      a. History and Physical
         (1) **Classic triad**
            (a) Lower abdominal pain
            (b) Amenorrhea
            (c) Irregular vaginal bleeding
         (2) Late changes (following rupture of tube)
            Signs and symptoms of an acute abdomen
      b. Laboratory
         (1) + β-hCG
         (2) Pelvic ultrasonography
            Can identify tubal implantation site *before* rupture occurs
   3. TREATMENT
      a. Surgery
         (1) Laparoscopy
         (2) Laparotomy

V. OVARY
   A. Benign ovarian tumors
   1. DEFINITION
      a. A benign neoplasm of the ovary.
      b. Histology
         (1) Epithelial cell
            (a) **Serous cystadenoma**
               ▸ The most common epithelial tumor
               ▸ 70% of all serous tumors are benign
               ▸ 15% are bilateral
               ▸ Most commonly present in perimenopausal or postmenopausal patients

(b) **Mucinous cystadenoma**
  ‣ The second most common epithelial tumor
  ‣ 85% of all mucinous tumors are benign
  ‣ 5% are bilateral
(2) Germ cell
  (a) Benign cystic teratoma (dermoid)
    ‣ Composed of differentiated tissues of embryonic germ layers
    ‣ Usually an asymptomatic cystic mass
    ‣ 10-20% are bilateral
    ‣ 99% of cystic teratomas are benign
(3) Sex cord tumors
  (a) Granulosa theca cell tumors
    ‣ **Functional tumors producing estrogenic hormones**
    ‣ Feminizing characteristics
    ‣ Have low-grade malignant potential
  (b) Sertoli-Leydig cell tumors
    ‣ **Functional tumors producing androgenic hormones**
    ‣ Virilizing characteristics
    ‣ Have low-grade malignant potential
  (c) Ovarian fibroma
    ‣ Meigs' syndrome
      • Ovarian fibroma + ascites + unilateral hydrothorax

2. DIAGNOSIS
  a. History and Physical
    (1) **Usually asymptomatic in early stages of the disease**
    (2) **Adnexal mass**
    (3) Nonspecific GI or GU complaints
    (4) Abdominal bloating or distention or pain
    (5) Irregular menses
    (6) Abnormal vaginal bleeding
    (7) ± abdominal mass
  b. Laboratory
    (1) **Tissue diagnosis obtained via surgery**
    (2) Ultrasonography
        Identifies solid, unilocular or complex masses
3. TREATMENT
  a. Cystectomy
  b. Unilateral oophorectomy
  c. Bilateral oophorectomy and hysterectomy

B. *Ovarian cancer*
   1. DEFINITION
     a. A primary malignancy of the ovary.
     b. Presents most commonly in the fifth and sixth decades of life
     c. Histology
       (1) Epithelial cell
         (a) ≈90% of all ovarian malignancies
         (b) **Serous cystadenocarcinoma**
           ▸ ≈ half of these tumors are derived from serous cystadenomas
           ▸ 30% are bilateral
         (c) **Mucinous cystadenocarcinoma**
           ▸ Can be huge tumors
           ▸ 10-15% bilateral
           ▸ Pseudomyxomatous peritonei
             Mucinous ascites
         (d) Endometrioid carcinoma
           ▸ Histologically similar to endometrial carcinoma
           ▸ May arise in conjunction with endometrial carcinoma
         (e) Clear cell
       (2) Germ cell
         (a) <5% of all ovarian malignancies
         (b) **Dysgerminoma**
           ▸ The most common ovarian cancer in women < 20 years of age
           ▸ 10-15% bilateral
           ▸ The most common germ cell tumor associated with gonadal dysgenesis
           ▸ It is the female equivalent to a seminoma
         (c) Immature teratoma
           ▸ Malignant equivalent to benign cystic teratoma
           ▸ Second most common germ cell tumor
           ▸ Usually associated with women <25 years of age
           ▸ ↑ of β-hCG and α-fetoprotein in mixed type tumors
         (d) Endodermal sinus tumor
           ▸ Rare tumors
           ▸ "Yolk sac" tumors
           ▸ Mean age of diagnosis is ≈18 years
           ▸ ↑ of α-fetoprotein

(e) Embryonal carcinoma
  ‣ Very rare
  ‣ Mean age of diagnosis is ≈14 years of age
  ‣ Secrete estrogen
  ‣ ↑ of β-hCG and α-fetoprotein
(f) Choriocarcinoma
  ‣ Extremely rare
  ‣ Usually diagnosed in patients <20 years if age
  ‣ Hormonally active
  ‣ ↑ of β-hCG
(3) Sex cord tumors
  (a) Granulosa-stromal cell tumors
    ‣ Low-grade malignancy
    ‣ **Functional tumors producing estrogenic hormones**
    ‣ Feminizing characteristics
  (b) Sertoli-Leydig cell tumors
    ‣ Usually a low-grade malignancy
    ‣ **Functional tumors producing androgenic hormones**
    ‣ Virilizing characteristics

2. DIAGNOSIS
  a. History and Physical
    (1) **Usually asymptomatic in early stages of the disease**
    (2) **Adnexal mass**
    (3) Nonspecific GI complaints
    (4) Abdominal pain
    (5) Abdominal bloating or distention
    (6) Irregular menses
    (7) Abnormal vaginal bleeding
    (8) Advanced disease
      ‣ Weight loss
      ‣ ± abdominal mass
      ‣ ± ascites
      ‣ Intestinal obstruction
  b. Laboratory
    (1) **Tissue diagnosis obtained via surgery**
    (2) Ultrasonography
       Identifies solid, unilocular or complex masses
    (3) Serum tumor markers
      (a) ↑ CA 125
        ‣ Usually used to *follow* the response to therapy

c. Staging
    (1) Stage I......Limited to the ovaries
    (2) Stage II....Cancer in one or both ovaries with extension to pelvic tissue
    (3) Stage III...Cancer in one or both ovaries with extension *outside* the pelvis (peritoneal implants) *and/or* + inguinal or retroperitoneal lymph nodes.
    (4) Stage IV...Distant metastases
d. **Surgical exploration**
    (1) Complex cyst by ultrasound
    (2) Persistent cyst by ultrasound
    (3) Any ovarian enlargement in postmenopausal women
    (4) A solid mass by ultrasound <8 cm in all premenopausal women
    (5) Any mass >8 cm in all premenopausal women
3. TREATMENT
  a. Epithelial tumors
    (1) Surgery
      (a) Total abdominal hysterectomy with bilateral salpingo-oophorectomy
      (b) Pelvic and para-aortic lymph node dissection
      (c) Tumor "debulking" procedures if necessary
    (2) Radiation therapy
      (a) Not indicated in *early* epithelial tumors
      (b) ± intraperitoneal radioactive phosphorus
      (c) Used *after* surgery and chemotherapy if tumor remains
    (3) Chemotherapy
      Cisplatin-based combination regimens
  b. Germ cell tumors
    (1) Surgery
      Unilateral or bilateral salpingo-oophorectomy
    (2) Radiation therapy
      (a) Dysgerminomas
        ↑ sensitive to radiation
      (b) Immature teratoma
        For localized disease following chemotherapy
    (3) Chemotherapy
      (a) Dysgerminoma
        Used when there is a primary treatment failure
      (b) Immature teratoma
        Indicated for advanced or high-grade lesions
      (c) Indicated in all other germ cell tumors

      c. Sex cord stromal tumors

          (1) Surgery

              (a) Simple oophorectomy for solitary mass

              (b) Total abdominal hysterectomy with bilateral salpingo-oophor-ectomy for involved disease

          (2) Radiation therapy

              Used when there is a primary treatment failure

          (3) Chemotherapy

              Used when there is a primary treatment failure

4. PROGNOSIS

      a. Five-year survival for *epithelial* tumors

          (1) Stage I...≈80%

          (2) Stage II..≈60%

          (3) Stage III...≈30%

          (4) Stage IV...≈ 5%

      b. Five-year survival for *germ cell* tumors

          (1) Dysgerminoma.......................................≈85-95%

          (2) Immature teratoma

               (a) Completely resected before chemotherapy........≈94%

              (b) Incompletely resected before chemotherapy......≈50%

          (3) Overall five-year survival for other *germ cell* tumors....≈60%

      c. Ten-year survival for *sex cord stromal* tumors..........................≈90%

VI. BREAST

    A. *Breast Abscess*

      1. DEFINITION

          a. An infection of the breast characterized by a localized accumulation of pus within the breast parenchyma.

          b. It can evolve from *mastitis*, an infection of the interlobar connective tissue of the breast.

          c. Etiologies

              (1) *Staphylococcus aureus*

              (2) *Streptococcus* spp.

      2. DIAGNOSIS

          a. History and Physical

              (1) **Breast pain**

              (2) **± painful breast mass**

              (3) Edema

              (4) Erythema

(5) ± fever

(6) ± axillary lymphadenopathy

(7) ± draining fistula

 b. Laboratory

  (1) CBC

   ↑ WBC count

  (2) Cultures

   To identify organism and check for antibiotic sensitivities

  (3) Mammograms and ultrasound if needed to evaluate the mass

3. TREATMENT

 a. Incise and drain the abscess

 b. Antibiotic therapy

  (1) Erythromycin

  (2) Cephalosporins

  (3) Amoxicillin/clavulanic acid

B. Galactorrhea

 1. DEFINITION

  a. A nipple discharge

  b. Galactorrhea + *normal menses* usually indicates a benign significance

  c. Etiologies

   (1) Functional

    (a) Drug induced

     ▸ Oral contraceptives

     ▸ Tricyclic antidepressants

     ▸ Phenothiazines

     ▸ Antihypertensives

     ▸ Reserpine

     ▸ ∝ Methyldopa

     ▸ Metoclopramide

     ▸ Cannabinoids

    (b) Organic

     ▸ Pituitary lesions

     ▸ Primary hypothyroidism

   (2) Serosanguinous/bloody

    (a) The majority are secondary to *benign* intraductal papilloma.

    (b) Cancer is present ≈ 10-15% of the time.

   (3) Postmenopausal

   Aggressive work-up to rule out cancer of the breast.

2. DIAGNOSIS
    a. History and physical
       See above
    b. Laboratory
       (1) ↑ serum prolactin level >300 ng/ml
          Usually associated with amenorrhea and pituitary disease
       (2) MRI
          Evaluation of the sella
       (3) Appropriate hormone studies to document endocrine disease
3. TREATMENT
    (1) Galactorrhea
       (a) Attempt to identify underlying cause and if it is drug induced
          discontinue it.
       (b) Pituitary microadenoma
          Bromocriptine ± surgery
       (c) Galactorrhea with *no* adenoma
          ▸ If the galactorrhea is tolerable → no treatment.
          ▸ Intolerable galactorrhea →Bromocriptine
    (2) Serosanguinous/Bloody
       Surgery to remove involved duct(s) and/or intraductal papilloma
C. *Fibrocystic Disease of the Breast*
    1. DEFINITION
       a. Fibrocystic disease is a misnomer. It is *not* a disease but an *exaggerated physiologic response* to fluctuating hormone levels in the body.
       b. **Fibrocystic change** is a term which encompasses an entire range of *benign breast diseases* which include:
          (1) **Nodularity, cysts and tumors**
             (a) Mastoplasia
                A change in the texture and consistency of the breast tissue which results in a thickening and nodularity of the breast.
            (b) Tumor
                ▸ Fibroadenoma
                   Average 1-3 cm tumor composed of proliferating epithelial and supporting fibrous tumors
            (c) Cysts
                A fluid-filled lesion within the breast parenchyma
          (2) **Mastalgia and engorgement**
            (a) Cyclic
                ↑ breast pain before menses which resolves with the onset or during menstruation.

      (b) Non-cyclic
- ▸ Benign breast lesions
  - • Duct ectasia
    - ○ May arise from chronic periductal and intra-inflammation
    - ○ Dilation of the ducts and inspissation of breast secretions
  - • Sclerosing adenosis
  - • Cysts
- ▸ Referred pain
  - • Chest wall
  - • Costochondritis
  - • Cardiovascular
  - • Neuritis

(3) **Nonproliferative lesions of the breast don't ↑ the risk of breast cancer**.
    (a) Fibroadenoma
    (b) Cysts
    (c) Mild hyperplasia

(4) **Proliferative lesions of the breast** *without atypia* **only slightly ↑ the risk of breast cancer**
    (a) Sclerosing adenosis
    (b) Intraductal papilloma
    (c) Moderate to severe hyperplasia

(5) **Atypical hyperplasia ↑ the risk of breast cancer and should be treated as a** *premalignant lesion*.

2. DIAGNOSIS
  a. History and Physical
    (1) The patient may be asymptomatic
    (2) *Breast pain and tenderness*
    (3) ± nipple discharge
    (4) ± breast mass
  b. Laboratory
    (1) Mammograms
      (a) Usually identifies the lesion
- ▸ **The mammogram is not infallible**
- ▸ 10-15% of breast cancers are *negative* on mammogram at the time of diagnosis

    (2) Ultrasound
    Differentiates solid and cystic lesions.

(3) Cytology

(a) Evaluation of aspirated fluid and cells from a cyst

(b) Evaluation of nipple discharge

↑ frequency of false negatives

(4) **Aspiration and/or needle biopsy**

(a) Evaluation of aspirated fluid and cells from a cyst

(b) Differentiates a solid and cystic lesions

(5) **Excisional biopsy**

Provides the histology (tissue diagnosis) of the lesion

(6) CT or MRI to identify pituitary lesions if galactorrhea is part of the differential diagnosis.

(7) ↑ serum prolactin level in galactorrhea

3. TREATMENT

a. Pain

(1) A well-fitted bra for support

(2) Local application of ice or heat

(3) Analgesics

(a) Acetaminophen

(b) NSAIDs

(4) Diet

(a) ↓ caffeine

(b) Vitamin E

(c) Vitamin B_6

(5) Spironolactone 7-10 days before menses

b. Nodularities

(1) Diet

(a) ↓ caffeine

(b) Surgical intervention if there is *any* question concerning a "lump" or nodularity.

c. Cysts

(1) Aspiration is usually curative.

(2) If cytology is negative routine follow up unless it recurs

(3) Aspiration of bloody fluid → surgical exploration

d. Tumors

See C.1.a. and C.2.a below

C. NEOPLASIA

1. *Fibroadenoma*

a. DEFINITION

(1) A *benign* breast tumor composed of both fibrous and glandular breast tissue.

(2) Most common breast tumor in young women.

(3) This lesion is important because it must be differentiated from breast cancer.

b. DIAGNOSIS

    (1) History and Physical

        (a) A painless, rubbery mass

        (b) Not fixed

        (c) Smooth regular borders

    (2) Laboratory

        (a) Mammogram

        (b) Ultrasound

            To differentiate cystic lesions from solid masses.

c. TREATMENT

    Surgical removal

2. *Breast Cancer*

a. DEFINITION

    (1) A primary malignancy of the breast.

    (2) High-risk factors

        (a) Family history

        (b) Age >40 years

        (c) Nulliparous

        (d) First pregnancy >30 years

        (e) Previous cancer in one breast

        (f) Atypical hyperplasia of the breast

    (3) Risk factors

        (a) Unopposed estrogens

        (b) ↑ fat diet

        (c) ↑ ETOH intake

        (d) Early menarche and late menopause

        (e) History of uterine, ovarian or colon cancer

        (f) Diabetes mellitus

    (4) Histology

        (a) **Ductal adenocarcinoma**.........≈**78%**

        (b) Lobular carcinoma.................≈ 9%

        (c) Comedocarcinoma.................≈ 5%

        (d) Medullary carcinoma..............≈ 4%

        (e) Colloid carcinoma.................≈ 3%

        (f) Inflammatory carcinoma...........≈ 1%

    (5) Breast cancer spreads by direct extension, blood and lymphatics

(6) Metastases
    (a) **Axillary lymph nodes**
    (b) Bone
    (c) Liver
    (d) Lung
    (e) Brain
(7) The presence of estrogen and progesterone receptors indicate a better prognosis and are necessary in deciding appropriate therapy.
(8) Negative axillary nodes at the time of surgery indicates a better prognosis

b. DIAGNOSIS
  (1) History and Physical
    (a) **Breast mass**
      ▸ Unilateral and hard
      ▸ Irregular, fixed and nontender
    (b) Nipple discharge
    (c) Peau d'orange
    (d) Nipple retraction
    (e) Dimpling
    (f) Axillary lymphadenopathy
  (2) Laboratory
    (a) Mammogram
    (b) Ultrasound
    (c) Aspiration and/or needle biopsy
    (d) Excisional biopsy
  (3) Physical exam + Mammograms + needle aspiration → a 93-100% detection
    (a) **If the lesion is malignant**
      ▸ CBC, Chem 28
      ▸ Chest X-ray
      ▸ CT of the abdomen
      ▸ Bone scan
      ▸ Liver scan if abnormal liver function studies
  (4) Staging
    (a) Stage 0..... Carcinoma In situ
    (b) Stage I......≤2 cm negative nodes
    (c) Stage II.....>2 cm and ≤5 cm, + nodes but *not* fixed
    (d) Stage IIIA.>5 cm, + nodes *fixed* to skin, chest wall or other axillary nodes

(e) Stage IIIB.Any size tumor, skin nodules or ulcerations, fixation of the tumor to the skin or chest wall or breast edema including peau d'orange + infraclavicular or supraclavcular nodes, arm edema ± palpable axillary nodes

(f) Stage IV....Distant metastases

c. TREATMENT

(1) There is great controversy concerning the treatment of breast cancer. Most discussion concerns treatment of stage I and II disease but opinions vary concerning all stages of disease.

(2) **Stage I and II disease**

(a) Modified radical mastectomy

(b) Lumpectomy + axillary node dissection for staging + Radiation therapy

(c) Chemotherapy

Combination drug therapy for six months

(d) Tamoxifen

▸ Premenopausal

• Tumors >1.0 cm, negative axillary nodes and, + hormone receptors

▸ Postmenopausal

• Tumors >1.0 cm and + hormone receptors

(e) Chemotherapy *is not indicated* for

▸ Carcinoma in situ

▸ Tumors <1.0 cm and negative nodes

(3) **Stage IIIA**

(a) Modified radical mastectomy followed by

(b) + hormone receptors and + axillary nodes

Radiation therapy + tamoxifen

(c) - hormone receptors and + axillary nodes

Chemotherapy and ± radiation therapy

(4) **Stage IIIB** (Inoperable)

(a) Chemotherapy x 3-4 months

(b) Radiation therapy followed by

(c) Modified radical mastectomy followed by

(d) Additional chemotherapy ± tamoxifen

(5) **Stage IV**

(a) Endocrine therapy

(b) Chemotherapy

         (c) Radiation therapy
- CNS and isolated bony metastases
- ↑ axillary metastases
  ± surgical resection

d. PROGNOSIS
    (1) Six-year survival
        (a) Stage O.................>98%
        (b) Stage I..................≈95%
        (c) Stage IIA..............≈84%
        (d) Stage IIB..............≈66%
        (e) Stage IIIA.............≈49%
        (f) Stage IIIB..............≈46%
        (g) Stage IV...............≈15%

I. DIAGNOSIS OF PREGNANCY
   A. Signs and symptoms
   1. *Cessation of menses*
   2. Nausea ± vomiting
   3. Breast tenderness and fullness
   4. Distention of the lower abdomen
   5. Fatigue
   B. Laboratory
   + β-hCG

II. INITIAL PRENATAL VISIT
   A. Complete History and Physical
   B. Laboratory
   1. Pap Smear
      Rule out any neoplastic lesions on the cervix
   2. CBC
      a. Evaluation of possible anemia
      b. Rule out any abnormalities of white blood cells
   3. Urinalysis ± culture
      a. Evaluate renal function
      b. Rule out infection
   4. Serum glucose
      Rule out diabetes mellitus
   5. Blood group and Rh factor
      a. Evaluate the risk of isoimmunization
      b. Blood typing and Rh status
   6. Indirect Coombs
      + antibody, identify the protein and manage patient to prevent hemolytic disease
   7. Sickle cell screen
      On all African-American patients
   8. Infectious disease screen
      a. PPD
         (1) If + then chest X-ray
         (2) If X-ray + then work up for TB, and begin treatment *after* delivery
      b. Rubella antibody titer
         (1) Test if immune status is unknown.
         (2) **Do not immunize during pregnancy.**

    c. Hepatitis B surface antigen

        If + treat infant with hepatitis B immune globulin and hepatitis B vaccine

    d. STD screen

        (1) Gonorrhea

        (2) Chlamydia

        (3) Syphilis

            Early diagnosis ↓ prenatal morbidity

    e. HIV

    f. High-risk patients

        Herpes simplex

9. Pelvic ultrasound

    If there is any discrepancy concerning dates

III. INTERVAL SCREENING

A. "Normal pregnancy"

    40 weeks ± 2 weeks calculated from the first day of the last menstrual cycle

B. A total weight gain of 28-30 pounds is ideal

C. Prenatal visits

    1. Every four weeks → 32 week of pregnancy

    2. Every two weeks → 36 week of pregnancy

    3. Every week until delivery

D. **First Trimester (up to 14 weeks)**

    1. Clinical assessment

        a. Blood pressure

        b. Urinalysis

        c. Uterine growth

        d. Maternal weight gain

        e. Detection of fetal heart beat by doppler ultrasound

        f. Genetic prenatal diagnostic testing

            (1) Early amniocentesis

            (2) Chorionic villous sampling

E. **Second Trimester (14-28 weeks)**

    1. History

        a. Review for obstetrical risk factors

            (1) Vaginal bleeding

            (2) Swelling of the face or hands

            (3) Continuous headache

            (4) Blurring of vision

            (5) Abdominal pain

            (6) Fever and chills

(7) Persistent vomiting

(8) Dysuria

(9) Escape of fluids from the vagina

(10) A change in intensity or frequency of fetal movement

2. Clinical assessment

    a. Blood pressure

    b. Urinalysis

    c. Quickening at 18-20 weeks

    d. Uterus at the umbilicus at 20 weeks

    e. Heart tones via stethoscope

    f. Check for gestational diabetes 24-28 weeks

    g. Serum $\propto$-fetoprotein

        Obtained at 16-20 weeks, it predicts open neural tube defects

    h. Ultrasonography

F. **Third Trimester (28 weeks to delivery)**

1. Review of obstetrical risk factors

    a. History

        (1) Vaginal bleeding

        (2) Swelling of the face or hands

        (3) Continuous headache

        (4) Blurring of vision

        (5) Abdominal pain

        (6) Fever and chills

        (7) Persistent vomiting

        (8) Dysuria

        (9) Escape of fluids from the vagina

        (10) A change in intensity or frequency of fetal movement

2. Clinical assessment

    a. Blood pressure

    b. Urinalysis

    c. Screen for anemia

        Hemoglobin and/or hematocrit

    d. Heart tones via stethoscope

    e. Check for gestational diabetes

    f. In high-risk patients recheck for STD

3. **A sudden weight gain in the third trimester is a warning sign of preeclampsia.**

4. Lightening

    $\approx$2-4 weeks before delivery the fetal head moves below the pubis symphysis

5. Cervical Effacement
    a. Softening and thinning of the cervix
    b. Loss of the mucous plug ("bloody show") and the beginning of labor.

IV. LABOR AND DELIVERY
  A. General
    1. Support and observation are the hallmarks of managing normal labor.
    2. Laboratory
      a. CBC
      b. Urinalysis
      c. Blood held for cross match
    3. IV placement
      a. Adequate fluids
      b. Use a 16-18 gauge venous catheter in case of possible emergency
    4. Appropriate analgesia
    5. Avoid the dorsal supine (lithotomy) position
      Compression of the inferior vena cava causing fetal and maternal distress.
  B. **First Stage**
    1. The onset of labor → full cervical dilation (10 cm)
    2. **Latent phase**
      a. A progressive dilation of the cervix with uterine contractions
      b. The duration is variable because of the time needed for cervical effacement.
      c. Latency ends with dilation of the cervix to 4 cm
    3. **Active phase**
      a. There are frequent, regular contractions
      b. The active phase ends with total cervical dilatation
    4. Fetal monitoring
      a. Low-risk = Every 15 minutes following contraction
      b. High-risk = Continuous
    5. Uterine contractions
      a. Low-risk = Every 30 minutes
      b. High-risk = Continuous
  C. **Second Stage**
    1. Full cervical dilation → delivery of the baby
    2. Fetal monitoring
      a. Low-risk = After every contraction
      b. High-risk = Continuous

3. **The cardinal movements of labor**
    a. Engagement
    b. Descent
    c. Flexion
    d. Internal rotation
    e. Extension
    f. External rotation
    g. Expulsion
4. The second stage ends with the birth of the baby

D. **Third Stage**
1. Delivery of the baby → delivery of the placenta
2. The placenta usually separates within 5-10 minutes
3. Once the placenta is delivered uterine massage and/or oxytocin IV

E. **Fourth Stage**
1. Delivery of the placenta → 2 hours postpartum
2. Postpartum uterine hemorrhage occurs about 1% of the time

V. APGAR SCORES

A. **Color**
1. Score
    a. 0 = Blue or pale all over
    b. 1 = Pink body, blue extremities
    c. 2 = Pink all over

B. **Heart rate**
1. Score
    a. 0 = Absent
    b. 1 = <100 beats per minute
    c. 2 = >100 beats per minute

C. **Respirations**
1. Score
    a. 0 = Absent
    b. 1 = Hypoventilation or weak cry
    c. 2 = Good effort or strong cry

D. **Muscle tone**
1. Score
    a. 0 = Absent
    b. 1 = Some flexion or motion
    c. 2 = Good flexion and motion

E. **Reflex irritability**
    1. Score
        a. 0 = Absent
        b. 1 = Grimace only
        c. 2 = Vigorous cry, sneeze or cough
F. Apgar scores are measured at 1 and 5 minutes
    1. At 1 minute
        a. Score <3
            Will probably need resuscitation
        b. Score 4-6
            Vigorous stimulation and/or brief respiratory support
        c. Score 7-10
            Will do well without special treatment
    2. At 5 minutes
        a. Scores <7 or falling
            (1) Indicates fetal distress.
            (2) The baby may be quite ill, requiring intensive care.

I. OSTEOMYELITIS
A. DEFINITION
1. An acute or chronic infection of bone usually caused by a bacteria or mycobacteria.
2. **Sequestra**

    Separation of bone in large fragments secondary to ischemic necrosis
3. **Involucrum**

    Deposition of new bone around the sequestra *after* the formation of subperiosteal or soft tissue abscesses
4. Classification and etiologies of osteomyelitis
    ### a. **Hematogenous osteomyelitis**
    (1) Most commonly diagnosed in
        - (a) Infants and children
        - (b) Older adults
        - (c) Injecting drug use
    (2) Accounts for ≈20% of cases
    (3) *Acute Hematogenous Osteomyelitis*
        - (a) Usually involves the long bones in the well-perfused metaphysis.
        - (b) Etiologies

            Staphylococcus aureus.............≈50% of cases
    (4) *Chronic Hematogenous Osteomyelitis*
        - (a) A relapse of acute osteomyelitis usually heralded by the presence of a non-healing ulcer or draining sinus tract.
        - (b) Lesion = bacteria + necrotic bone + compromised soft tissue surrounding it.
        - (c) Etiology

            Mixed bacterial infections
        - (d) <5% of cases of acute hematogenous osteomyelitis progress to chronic osteomyelitis
    (5) *Vertebral Osteomyelitis*
        - (a) Usually occurs in adults secondary to a bacteremia
            - ▸ Urinary tract
            - ▸ Endocarditis
            - ▸ Soft tissue infection
            - ▸ Contaminated IV line
            - ▸ Injecting drug use
        - (b) Most often hematogenous but *may* be secondary to trauma.
        - (c) Etiologies
            - ▸ *E coli and Salmonella* sp......≈30% of cases
            - ▸ *Pseudomonas aeruginosa* and *Serratia* sp.
                - • Injecting drug use

> ‣ *Staphylococcus aureus* and *Salmonella* spp.
>> • Sickle cell anemia and other hemoglobinopathies
> ‣ *Mycobacterium tuberculosis*
>> • **Pott's disease**
>>> Tuberculous spondylitis most commonly involving the thoracic spine

b. **Contiguous Focus Osteomyelitis**
  (1) With no generalized vascular insufficiency
    (a) ↑ number of cases in adults
    (b) Most commonly associated with
      ‣ Penetrating injuries
      ‣ Surgical procedures
      ‣ Direct extension of infection from surrounding soft tissues
    (c) Etiologies
      ‣ *Staphylococcus aureus* isolated most often but mixed bacterial infections occur.
      ‣ *Pseudomonas aeruginosa*
        Puncture wound of the foot or thermal burns
      ‣ *Pasteurella multocida*
        Animal bites
  (2) With generalized vascular insufficiency
    a. Almost always associated with adult diabetics
      ‣Most commonly associated with the small bones of the feet.
      ‣ Diabetic neuropathy → trauma → soft tissue infection → compromised circulation → infection.
    b. Etiologies
      ‣ *Staphylococcus aureus*
      ‣ *Staphylococcus epidermidis*
      ‣ Anaerobic infection

B. DIAGNOSIS
  1. History and Physical
    a. Hematogenous osteomyelitis
      (1) Fever
      (2) Lethargy
      (3) Pain in the area of the infection
      (4) Soft tissue inflammation surrounding the lesion
    b. Vertebral osteomyelitis
      (1) ± fever
      (2) Point tenderness over the lesion

(3) Neck or back pain

   c. Contiguous focus osteomyelitis

      (1) Pain over the lesion

      (2) Erythema

      (3) Tenderness

      (4) ± draining sinus or ulcer

  2. Laboratory

    a. Needle aspiration or biopsy of bony lesion

      (1) The *definitive test* for diagnosis

        (a) Gram stain

        (b) Culture and sensitivity

    b Blood cultures

      + cultures ≈50% of the time with hematogenous osteomyelitis

    c. CBC

      ↑ WBCs in acute cases

    d. ↑ sedimentation rate

    e. X-rays

      (1) Hematogenous osteomyelitis

        (a) Initial

          Soft tissue swelling

        (b) Early (≈10 days)

          Periosteal reaction

        (c) Late changes (2-6 weeks)

          Lytic changes

      (2) Vertebral osteomyelitis

        (a) Irregular erosions in the end plates of adjacent vertebral bodies

        (b) ↓ intervening disk space

      (3) Contiguous focus osteomyelitis

        May not be able to distinguish from underlying infection

    f. Bone scan

      + within 24 hours of symptoms

    g. CT or MRI

      Lesions can be identified *very* early in the course of disease

C. TREATMENT

  1. General

    a. Antibiotic therapy is dependent upon organism(s) isolated

    b. Treatment lasts 4-6 weeks

2. Hematogenous
   a. Empiric therapy
      (1) *Staphylococcus aureus*
         (a) Oxacillin
         (b) Nafcillin
         (c) Cephalosporin
         (d) Vancomycin
      (2) Gram-negatives
         (a) Third-generation cephalosporin
         (b) Aminoglycosides
         (c) Fluoroquinolones
   b. Surgery is indicated if
      (1) Soft tissue abscess
      (2) Infected joint
      (3) If no response to antibiotics in 48 hours
3. Contiguous focus/Chronic osteomyelitis
   a. Surgery
      (1) Debridement
      (2) Removal of prosthetic joint
   b. Antibiotic therapy
      Dependent upon organism(s) isolated

II. ARTHRITIS
   A. *Rheumatoid Arthritis*
      1. DEFINITION
         a. Rheumatoid arthritis is a disease of unknown etiology characterized by a symmetrical inflammatory polyarthritis.
         b. Rheumatoid arthritis can affect *any* diarthrodial joint.
            (1) Joint involvement (By frequency)
               (a) Small joints of the hands
               (b) Wrists
               (c) Knees
               (d) Feet
               (e) Elbows
               (f) Shoulders
               (g) Hips
               (h) Ankles
         c. **The characteristic finding is a persistent inflammatory synovitis.**
         d. Joint involvement is usually symmetrical

2. DIAGNOSIS
    a. American Rheumatology Association criteria for diagnosis. (4 of 7 criteria)
    b. Criteria 1-4 must be present for six weeks and must be confirmed by a physician
        (1) Morning stiffness (≥ 1 hour)
        (2) Soft tissue swelling of three or more joints
        (3) Soft tissue swelling of hand joints
            (a) Proximal interphalangeal (PIP)
            (b) Metacarpophalangeal (MCP)
            (c) Wrist
        (4) Symmetric soft tissue swelling
        (5) Subcutaneous nodules
            Usually periarticular on extensor surfaces
        (6) Serum rheumatoid factor
        (7) Erosions and/or periarticular osteopenia on X-ray
            (a) Hand
            (b) Wrist
    c. Constitutional signs and symptoms
        (1) Fatigue
        (2) Malaise
        (3) $\pm$ Fever
    d. Extra-articular disease
        (1) Skin
        (2) Eyes
        (3) Lungs
        (4) Heart and blood vessels
        (5) Nervous system.
    e. Laboratory
        (1) CBC
            Normocytic, normochromic anemia
        (2) ↑ sedimentation rate
        (3) + rheumatoid factor $\approx 80\%$ of the cases
        (4) Synovial fluid analysis
            (a) Cloudy yellow fluid
            (b) Poor mucin clot
            (c) WBCs = 3000-50,000 cells/mm^3
            (d) Complement is low

3. TREATMENT
    a. Nonpharmacologic
        (1) Rest
        (2) Appropriate exercise

(3) Physical therapy

(4) Occupational therapy

b. Pharmacologic

    (1) NSAIDs

    (2) Disease-modifying antirheumatic drugs

        (a) Gold compounds

        (b) Sulfasalazine

        (c) Hydroxychloroquine

        (d) D-penicillamine

    (3) Glucocorticoid therapy

        (a) Intra-articular steroid injection

        (b) Avoid *if* possible because of long-term toxicity

            ‣ ± monthly pulses with high-dose corticosteroids

            ‣ ± low-dose prednisone

    (4) Immunosuppressive therapy

        (a) Methotrexate

        (b) Azathioprine

        (c) Cyclophosphamide

    (5) Surgery

        Joint replacement

B. *Osteoarthritis (Degenerative Joint Disease)*

    1. DEFINITION

        a. Osteoarthritis, the *most common* rheumatic disease

        b. There is *progressive loss* of articular cartilage followed by bone remodeling and bony overgrowth of the diarthrodial (movable, synovial-lined) joint(s).

        c. Osteoarthritis may be primary or secondary

            (1) Primary

                (a) Idiopathic

                    "Aging" and not related to systemic or local disease

            (2) Secondary

                (a) Post-traumatic

                (b) Congenital

                    Bone dysplasias

                (c) Metabolic

                    ‣ Hemoglobinopathies

                    ‣ Wilson's disease

                (d) Endocrine

                    ‣ Hyperparathyroidism

                    ‣ Acromegaly

                    ‣ Hypothyroidism

(e) Inflammatory

Septic arthritis

2. DIAGNOSIS

a. History and Physical

(1) Early joint disease

(a) **Joint pain**

(b) ↓ range of motion

(c) Morning stiffness

(d) ± joint thickening

(e) ± effusion

(2) Late joint disease

(a) Joint instability

(b) Pain at rest which ↑ with movement and weight bearing.

(3) Hands

(a) The *most common location* of osteoarthritis

(b) Heberden's nodes

Bony enlargement of the *distal* interphalangeal joints.

(c) Bouchard's nodes

Bony enlargement of the *proximal* interphalangeal joints.

b. Laboratory

(1) There are no specific laboratory tests for osteoarthritis.

(2) Remember, the sedimentation rate is usually normal

(3) Synovial fluid examination

(a) Normal color/viscosity

(b) Negative mucin clot test

(c) WBCs = 150-1500 cells/mm³

(d) Wear and mineral particles

(4) X-rays

(a) Early

Normal

(b) Late

‣ ↓ joint space

‣ Osteophyte formation

‣ Subchondral bony sclerosis

‣ Bony cysts in subchondral or denuded bone.

(5) CT/MRI

Important in evaluation of spinal osteoarthritis.

3. TREATMENT

a. Nonpharmacologic

(1) Moderate activity

(2) ↑ joint rest

(3) Joint protection

Walkers, canes etc.

(4) Weight reduction in the overweight

(5) Hot or cold packs

(6) Physical therapy

b. Pharmacologic

(1) Analgesics

(2) NSAIDs

▸ Beware of peptic ulcer disease as a side effect

Caution especially over the age of 60

(3) Muscle relaxants

(4) Intra-articular steroid injection

(5) Surgery

(a) By arthroscope

Debridement and repair

(b) Joint replacement

(6) **Systemic steroids have no role in the treatment of osteoarthritis**.

III. SYSTEMIC LUPUS ERYTHEMATOSUS

A. DEFINITION

1. A disease of unknown etiology that primarily affects women of child bearing age.

2. It is characterized by a multisystem autoimmune inflammatory response.

Antibodies react with nuclear, cytoplasmic and cell membrane antigens.

3. Lupus may be relatively benign or follow a fulminant course with involvement of the kidneys and central nervous system resulting in death.

4. The disease is marked by exacerbations and remissions.

B. DIAGNOSIS

1. American Rheumatology Association criteria for diagnosis.

4 of 11 criteria simultaneously or serially.

a. Malar "butterfly" rash

b. Discoid rash

c. Photosensitivity

d. Ulcerations

(1) Oral

(2) Nasopharyngeal

e. Nonerosive arthritis

≥2 peripheral joints

f. Serositis

(1) Pleuritis *or*

(2) Pericarditis

g. Renal disorder

(1) Proteinuria *or*

(2) Cellular casts

h. Neurologic disorder

(1) Seizures *or*

(2) Psychosis

i. Hematologic disorder

(1) Hemolytic anemia *with* reticulocytosis *or*

(2) Leukopenia *or*

<4000 cells/mm³ x2

(3) Lymphopenia *or*

<1500 cells/mm³ x2

(4) Thrombocytopenia *or*

$<100,000$/mm³

j. Immunologic disorder

(1) + LE cell prep *or*

(2) + Anti-DNA *or*

Antibody to native DNA

(3) + Anti-Sm *or*

Antibody to Sm nuclear antigen

(4) False + serologic test for syphilis

k. Antinuclear antibody

2. Patients may also exhibit

a. Fatigue

b. Fever

c. Weight loss

d. Arthralgias

3. Laboratory

a. Serum antibodies in ↑ titers

(1) ANA

Screening

(2) **dsDNA and Sm antibodies**

b. Hematologic

(1) CBC

(a) **Anemia**

(b) Leukopenia $\approx 50\%$ of patients

c. Renal

(1) Proteinuria

(2) Casts

(3) WBCs

d. Hypergammaglobulinemia

C. TREATMENT

1. General

a. Adequate rest

b. ↓ stress

c. ↑ exercise

2. Photosensitivity

a. Sun-screens/block

b. Topical steroids

c. Intralesional injections of steroids for resistant lesions

d. Refractory cases

(1) Hydroxychloroquine

(2) Systemic steroids (last resort)

3. Arthritis/Pleuritis/pericarditis

a. NSAIDs

b. Systemic steroids

4. Nephritis

a. Proteinuria + normal renal function

Systemic steroids

b. If renal insufficiency occurs

(1) Kidney biopsy

(2) Therapy is dependent upon the glomerular lesion

(a) IV cyclophosphamide

(b) ± prednisone

c. Renal failure

(1) Dialysis

5. Central nervous system

a. Seizures

See Chapter 13, Neurology II.A.1.

b. Encephalitis

(1) Systemic steroids

6. Hematologic

a. Hemolysis

(1) Systemic steroids

(2) Failure of therapy

(a) Immunosuppressive therapy

(b) Splenectomy

b. Thrombocytopenia

Systemic steroids

I. DIABETES MELLITUS

A. DEFINITION

1. A disease characterized by *hypoinsulinemia* yielding
    a. Hyperglycemia
    b. Glucose intolerance
2. Classification
    a. **Insulin-dependent diabetes mellitus (Type I)**
        (1) The etiology is unknown
            (a) Circulating islet cell antibodies destroy the capability of the pancreas to produce insulin.
            (b) Anti-insulin and anti-islet antibodies are frequently present years before onset of diabetes.
            (c) There *is* an HLA association.
        (2) Incidence
            Usually <30 years with a peak at 11-13 years but can occur at any age
        (3) *Ketosis occurs frequently*
        (4) Insulin-dependent diabetes mellitus represents ≈10% of all cases.
    b. **Non-insulin-dependent diabetes mellitus (Type II)**
        (1) Non-insulin-dependent diabetes mellitus represents ≈90% of all cases
        (2) *Ketosis rarely occurs.*
        (3) Usually >40 years at diagnosis
        (4) Insulin secretion is *variable* ranging from a moderate deficiency to hyperinsulinemia.
        (5) Insulin resistance is usual

B. DIAGNOSIS

1. History and Physical
    a. **Polydipsia**
    b. **Polyphagia**
    c. **Polyuria**
    d. **Fatigue**
    e. Blurring of vision
    f. ± weight loss
    g. ± weakness
    h. ± infection
2. Laboratory
    a. Criteria for the diagnosis of diabetes in nonpregnant adults
        (1) Fasting venous plasma glucose ≥140 mg/dL x2 *or*
        (2) Following ingestion of 75 grams of glucose, *two* venous plasma glucose readings of ≥200 mg/dL, with one of the readings taken at two hours.
        (3) Random glucose >200 mg/dL + polyuria, polydipsia, and polyphagia

C. TREATMENT
   1. General
      a. Diet
         (1) Based on an appropriate number of calories for the patient's body weight
         (2) Low in saturated fat and cholesterol
         (3) Adequate protein intake balanced with 50-60% carbohydrates
      b. Exercise
   2. Insulin-dependent diabetes mellitus
      a. **Treatment with insulin is always required.**
         (1) Insulin regimens must be tailored to the patient
         (2) Insulin protocols
            (a) Mixed or split program
               NPH or lente insulin + regular insulin mixed and given in the morning and evening
            (b) Three-injection program
               ▸ NPH or lente insulin pre-breakfast
               ▸ Regular insulin pre-supper
               ▸ NPH or lente insulin at bedtime
            (c) Ultralente-regular program
               ▸ Ultralente insulin twice daily
               ▸ Regular insulin before each meal
   3. Non-insulin-dependent diabetes mellitus
      a. If diet and exercise do not ↓ the blood sugar to normal add an *oral hypoglycemic*
         (1) Sulfonylureas
            (a) Glyburide
            (b) Glipizide
         (2) Some patients *may* require insulin
   4. Monitoring of blood glucose
      a. Home monitoring of glucose once or twice daily is essential
      b. *Glycosylated hemoglobin*
         (1) Assess long-term control
         (2) It reflects an estimate of blood glucose for the preceding 3-months
   5. Goals for control of blood glucose
      a. Fasting
         (1) Ideal...................70-100 mg/dL
         (2) Acceptable.........60-130 mg/dL
      b. One hour postprandial
         (1) Ideal.................... <200 mg/dL
         (2) Acceptable...........<160 mg/dL

II. PITUITARY DISEASE

A. *Acromegaly* and *Gigantism*

1. DEFINITION

    a. Diseases characterized by an increased level of growth hormone

    (1) **Acromegaly**

    An increase in growth hormone occurs *after* epiphyseal closure

    (2) **Gigantism**

    An increase in growth hormone occurs *before* epiphyseal closure

2. DIAGNOSIS

    a. History and physical (acromegaly)

    (1) **Acral enlargement**

    (2) **Soft tissue overgrowth**

    (3) **Fatigue**

    (4) Hyperhidrosis

    (5) Weight gain

    (6) Joint pain

    (7) Parathesias

    (8) Irregular or absent menses

    (9) ↓ libido

    (10) Headache

    (11) Hypertension

    (12) Glucose intolerance

    (13) ↑ size of tongue

    b. Laboratory

    (1) Measurement of growth hormone

    (a) Basal level usually >5 μg/L

    Not useful for screening

    (2) Glucose-suppressed growth hormone determination

    Growth hormone levels will not be suppressed <2 μg/L

    (3) IGF-I plasma measurement

    This mediator of growth hormone is elevated

    (4) X-ray

    Coned-down view of sella turcica is abnormal in 90% of patients

    (5) MRI or CT

    Excellent for diagnosis and therapeutic planning

3. TREATMENT

    a. Surgery

    Transsphenoidal surgery

    b. Radiation therapy

    Pituitary radiation

III. **THYROID DISEASE**
    A. *Hypothyroidism*
        1. DEFINITION
            a. An illness characterized by a deficiency of thyroid hormone.
            b. Etiologies
                (1) *Primary hypothyroidism*
                    (a) A *primary* thyroid gland failure responsible for ≈90% of disease
-     ▸ Congenital
-     ▸ Acquired
  - • Post-surgical
  - • Treatment with radioactive iodine
  - • **Hashimoto's thyroiditis**
    - ◦ Chronic lymphocytic thyroiditis
    - ◦ Women >50 years of age
    - ◦ Diffuse goiter
    - ◦ + antithyroid antibodies
-     ▸ Abnormal thyroid function
  - • Endemic goiter
    - ◦ Iodine deficiency
    - ◦ Goitrogens
-     ▸ Drug-induced
  - • Iodine
  - • Lithium carbonate
  - • Amiodarone

                (2) *Secondary hypothyroidism*
                    (a) A failure of the hypothalamic-pituitary axis
-     ▸ Hypothalamic lesion
  - • ↓ Thyroid *Releasing* Hormone (TRH)
-     ▸ Pituitary lesion
  - • ↓ Thyroid *Stimulating* Hormone (TSH)

                (3) Tissue resistance to thyroid hormone
                (4) **Subclinical hypothyroidism**
                    (a) Normal T_4 but ↑ TSH
                        These patients should be treated with levothyroxine and fol-
                        lowed by serial monitoring of the TSH which should return to a
                        normal level with therapy.

        2. DIAGNOSIS
            a. History and Physical
                (1) General
                    (a) **Fatigue**

(b) **Weight gain**

(c) **Cold intolerance**

(d) **Weakness**

(e) Dull, expressionless face

(f) Eyelid droop

(g) Deep, hoarse voice

(2) Integument and subcutaneous tissues

(a) $\downarrow$ hair

(b) Coarse, cool skin

(c) Periorbital puffiness

(d) Swelling of hands

(e) Myxedema

A hydrophilic mucopolysaccharide that accumulates in subcutaneous tissues in *severe* disease.

(3) Cardiovascular

(a) Bradycardia

(b) Cardiomegaly

(4) Gastrointestinal

(a) Constipation

(b) Macroglossia

(5) Gynecological

Menorrhagia

(6) Musculoskeletal

(a) Stiffness and cramping of muscles

(b) Carpal tunnel syndrome

(7) Neurological

(a) Prolongation of tendon reflex contraction and relaxation

(b) Parathesias

(c) $\downarrow$ Memory

(8) Psychiatric

Depression

b. Laboratory

(1) $\downarrow$ serum T_4 in all cases of hypothyroidism

(2) TSH is $\uparrow$ in primary hypothyroidism

(3) TSH is $\downarrow$ or normal in secondary hypothyroidism

(4) CBC

Anemia

(5) Chem 28

(a) $\uparrow$ cholesterol

(b) $\uparrow$ creatinine phosphokinase

(6) ECG

    (a) Bradycardia

    (b) ↓ amplitude of QRS

    (c) Inverted or flattened T waves

3. TREATMENT

    a. Levothyroxine

        (1) 25 micrograms initially and advance by 25-50 micrograms every 3-4 weeks.

        (2) Monitor replacement therapy with serum T_3, T_4 and TSH levels until normalized

        (3) With secondary hypothyroidism, do not give thyroxine until adrenal insufficiency has been treated.

B. *Hyperthyroidism (Thyrotoxicosis)*

    1. DIAGNOSIS

        a. An illness characterized by an excess level of circulating thyroid hormone.

        b. Thyrotoxicosis

            (1) Graves' Disease

                (a) responsible for ≈85% of cases

                (b) An autoimmune disease characterized by the presence of IgG class *Thyroid Stimulating Immunoglobulin* that bind to the TSH receptors in the thyroid gland and stimulate the gland to produce ↑ levels of T_3 and T_4.

                (c) Two manifestations not found in other types of hyperthyroidism

                    ▸ Pretibial myxedema

                    ▸ Exophthalmos

            (2) Toxic multinodular goiter

                (a) Common in older patients

                (b) May be precipitated by iodine-containing drugs

            (3) Toxic adenoma

            (4) Subacute thyroiditis

                Painful goiter + transient, mild hyperthyroidism

    2. DIAGNOSIS

        a. History and Physical

            (1) Thyroid

                ± enlargement

            (2) General

                (a) Heat intolerance

                (b) Nervousness

                (c) ↑ sweating

                (d) Weight loss

                (e) Fatigue and weakness

(3) Integument
    (a) Palmar erythema
    (b) Warm, moist skin
    (c) Pretibial myxedema
(4) Cardiovascular
    (a) Palpitations
    (b) Tachycardia
    (c) Widened pulse pressure
(5) Respiratory
    Dyspnea
(6) Gastrointestinal
    (a) ↑ frequency of bowel movements
    (b) ↑ appetite
(7) Gynecological
    (a) Amenorrhea
    (b) Oligomenorrhea
(8) Neurological
    (a) Ophthalmologic
        ▸ Lid lag on downward gaze
        ▸ ↓ blinking
        ▸ ↑ widening of the palpebral fissures
        ▸ Stare
    (b) Ophthalmopathy
        ▸ ± ophthalmoplegia
        ▸ Periorbital swelling
        ▸ Conjunctivitis
        ▸ Exophthalmos
        ▸ Chemosis
    (c) Fine tremor
(9) Psychiatric
    (a) Emotional lability
    (b) Insomnia
c. Laboratory
    (1) ↓ TSH < 0.1 μU/ml
    (2) ↑ T_4 >12.5 μg/dL
        (a) T_4 **is almost totally protein bound to thyroxine-binding globulin (TBG).**
        (b) TBG is ↑ with
            ▸ Pregnancy
            ▸ Estrogen

▸ Liver disease

(3) ↑ T_3 (RIA) >200 ng/mL.

(4) FTI (Free Thyroxine Index) >12

(5) Radioactive iodine uptake

    (a) ↑ Graves' disease

    (b) ± ↑ in toxic nodules

(6) ECG

    (a) Sinus tachycardia

    (b) Atrial fibrillation

3. TREATMENT

  a. Radioactive iodine

    (1) Results in thyroid tissue ablation

    (2) Requires thyroid hormone replacement therapy

  b. Subtotal thyroidectomy

    (1) For patients with contraindications to radioactive iodine

      Pregnancy

    (2) ± thyroid replacement therapy

  c. Antithyroid medications

    (1) PTU (propylthiouracil)

    (2) Propranolol to control the tachycardia

    (3) Diltiazem if propranolol is contraindicated

C. *Thyroid cancer*

  1. DEFINITION

    a. A primary malignancy of the thyroid gland

    b. Histologic typing and biologic behavior

      (1) **Papillary carcinoma**...**≈70% of cases**

        (a) Affect younger population

        (b) Psammoma bodies present

        (c) + regional lymph nodes in half the cases

        (d) Distant metastases occur late

        (e) ↑ risk following radiation exposure

      (2) Follicular carcinoma.....................................≈20% of cases

        (a) Peak incidence at 40 years of age

        (b) They metastasize hematogenously

        (c) ↑ risk with iodine deficiency

      (3) Anaplastic giant cell/Spindle cell carcinoma.................≈5% of cases

        (a) Affect patients >60 years of age

        (b) An aggressive tumor

(4) Medullary carcinoma...≈ 5% of cases
        (a) They can be hormonally active
            ‣ ACTH
            ‣ Histaminase
            ‣ Calcitonin
        (b) Amyloid may be present
        (c) Metastases late in the course of disease

2. DIAGNOSIS
    a. History and Physical
        (1) ↑ **neck mass**
        (2) Hoarseness
        (3) Neck pain
        (4) Dysphagia
        (5) ± cervical lymphadenopathy
    b. Laboratory
        (1) Thyroid scan
            (a) **"Cold nodules"**
                ‣ These lesions are nonfunctional are present 90% of the time in patients with palpable thyroid nodules.
                ‣ **Only ≈10% will be malignant**
        (2) Ultrasound
            (a) Will not differentiate benign from malignant lesions
            (b) Will differentiate solid and cystic lesions
            (c) Malignancies are more likely to be solid lesions
        (3) Fine needle biopsy
            (a) **Excellent method for diagnosis**
            (b) 90% accurate for benign lesions
            (c) 60-70% accurate for malignant lesions
        (4) Open biopsy
            Used when the needle biopsy is suspicious but not diagnostic

3. TREATMENT
    a. Surgery
        Total or near-total thyroidectomy
    b. Thyroxine
        To suppress TSH and keep patient euthyroid
    c. Radioactive iodine
        (1) Results in thyroid tissue ablation
        (2) Requires thyroid hormone replacement therapy

4. PROGNOSIS
    a. Ten-year survival
        (1) Papillary carcinoma
            (a) <40 years of age.............................≈95%
            (b) >40 years of age.............................≈75%
        (2) Follicular carcinoma
            (a) Without vascular invasion.................≈95%
            (b) With vascular invasion.....................≈35%
        (3) Medullary carcinoma
            (a) - lymph nodes................................≈95%
            (b) + lymph nodes (five-year)................≈45%
        (4) Anaplastic carcinoma
            Most patients die within 6-8 months of diagnosis

IV. PARATHYROID DISEASE
    A. *Hypoparathyroidism*
        1. DEFINITION
            a. A disease characterized by a ↓ PTH level and/or action which may result in *hypocalcemia* and *hyperphosphatemia*.
            b. Etiologies
                (1) Idiopathic
                    (a) Congenital absence
                    (b) Autoimmune
                (2) Acquired
                    (a) Surgical removal during thyroidectomy or other neck surgery
                    (b) Radiation
        2. DIAGNOSIS
            a. History and Physical
                (1) Integument
                    (a) Skin dryness
                    (b) Brittle nails
                (2) Eyes
                    Cataracts
                (3) Cardiovascular
                    Arrhythmias
                (4) Neuromuscular
                    (a) Dysphagia
                    (b) ↑ DTRs
                    (c) Carpopedal spasm
                    (d) Chvostek's sign

           (e) Tetany

        (5) Psychiatric

           (a) Organic brain syndrome

           (b) Psychosis

    b. Laboratory

        (1) ↓ total serum calcium (<8.4 mg/dL)

        (2) ↑ serum phosphate

        (3) ↓ PTH

3. TREATMENT

    a. Tetany

        IV calcium gluconate

    b. Chronic hypocalcemia

        (1) Vitamin D

        (2) Oral calcium

B. *Hyperparathyroidism*

  1. DEFINITION

    a. A disease characterized by an ↑ PTH level which elevates the serum calcium >10.2 mg/dL.

    b. **Primary hyperparathyroidism**

        (1) **Single adenoma...............≈80% of the time**

        (2) Hyperplasia......................≈15% of the time

        (3) Multiple adenomas.............≈5% of the time

    c. **Secondary hyperparathyroidism**

        (1) Chronic renal failure

        (2) Malabsorption

        (3) Vitamin D deficiency

        (4) Pregnancy

    d. **Parathyroid carcinoma is rare.**

  2. DIAGNOSIS

    a. >90% of patients an ↑ serum calcium have primary hyperparathyroidism or a malignancy.

    b. History and Physical

        (1) General

           (a) Fatigue

           (b) Weight loss

           (c) Weakness

        (2) Musculoskeletal

           (a) Muscle weakness

           (b) Bony pain

           (c) Cystic bone lesions

           (d) Arthralgias

           (e) Fractures

     (3) Gastrointestinal

           (a) Anorexia

           (b) Nausea and vomiting

           (c) Abdominal pain

           (d) Constipation

           (e) Pancreatitis

     (4) Kidney

           (a) Kidney stones

           (b) Nephrocalcinosis

     (5) Psychiatric

           (a) Anxiety/depression

           (b) Psychosis

  c. Laboratory

     (1) ↑ total serum calcium (>10.2 mg/dL x3)

     (2) ↑ PTH

     (3) ↓ serum phosphate (<2.5 mg/dL)

     (4) X-ray

        Osteopenia in primary hyperparathyroidism

3. TREATMENT

  a. Primary

     Surgery

  b. Secondary

     (1) If possible correct the underlying illness

     (2) ± surgery

     (3) Medical management by manipulation of the serum calcium and phosphate

           (a) Hydration

           (b) ↑ salt intake

           (c) Furosemide

           (d) Glucocorticoids

           (e) Oral/IV phosphate

           (f) Biphosphonates

           (g) Mithramycin

           (h) Calcitonin

     (4) Dialysis

V. ADRENAL DISEASE
    A. Adrenocortical Insufficiency
        1. DEFINITION
            a. A disorder characterized by a deficiency of cortisol ± a deficiency of aldosterone
            b. Primary adrenal insufficiency
                (1) **Addison's disease**
                    ▸ A disease or disorder of the *adrenal glands* causing ↓ cortisol
                    ▸ Most common etiologies
                        • Autoimmune adrenalitis
                        • Hemorrhage
            c. Secondary adrenal insufficiency
                (1) A deficiency of ACTH caused by a hypothalamic-pituitary insufficiency
                (2) Most common etiologies
                    ▸ Discontinuance of longstanding exogenous glucocorticoid therapy
                    ▸ Pituitary or hypothalamic tumors
        2. DIAGNOSIS
            a. History and physical
                (1) Fatigue
                (2) Weight loss
                (3) Unexplained weight loss
                (4) Orthostatic hypotension
                (5) Anorexia
                (6) Nausea and vomiting
                (7) Diarrhea
                (8) Fasting hypoglycemia
                (9) Dilutional hyponatremia
            b. In addition with patients with primary adrenal insufficiency
                (1) Hyponatremia and hyperkalemia
                    Loss of aldosterone
                (2) Loss of axillary and pubic hair
                    Loss of adrenal androgens
                (3) Hyperpigmentation over palmar creases and extensor surfaces
                    ACTH which has a melanocyte-stimulating effect and is elevated
            c. In addition with patients with secondary adrenal insufficiency
                (1) Pallor
                (2) Sun sensitivity
             d. Laboratory
                (1) Measurement of
                    (a) 0800-hour plasma cortisol <10 μg/dL or
                    (b) 24-hour urinary free cortisol <50 μg

(2) If clinically suspect or screening values are low then

(3) Cortrosyn stimulation test

Detects both primary and secondary adrenal insufficiency

(4) CT or MRI of the adrenals and/or pituitary gland

3. TREATMENT

a. If possible, treat the underlying disease or disorder

b. Replacement therapy

(1) Hydrocortisone or

(2) Cortisone acetate or

(3) Prednisone

c. Primary adrenal insufficiency

(1) Mineralocorticoid replacement

Fludrocortisone

B. *Cushing's Syndrome*

1. DEFINITION

a. A syndrome(s) caused by ↑ exposure to glucocorticoid hormone excess.

(1) Exogenous

(a) Iatrogenic

▸ Extended treatment with glucocorticoids or ACTH

▸ A common cause of Cushings syndrome

(2) Endogenous

(a) ↑ secretion of corticotropin-releasing hormone

(b) ↑ secretion of ACTH

(c) ↑ secretion of cortisol

b. Endogenous Cushing's syndrome

(1) ACTH-dependent..≈80-85%

(a) **Cushing's disease**

▸ The *pituitary* produces ↑ ACTH......................≈80%

▸ Comprises ≈65% of all Cushing's disease

▸ ≈95% have corticotrop-secreting pituitary adenomas

(b) Nonpituitary lesions

Corticotropin-releasing hormone or ACTH........≈20%

(2) ACTH-independent..≈15%

The majority are caused by adrenocortical neoplasms

2. DIAGNOSIS

a. History and Physical

(1) Rounded face

(2) Reddish-purple striae

(3) Fat deposits over posterior neck

(4) Proximal muscle weakness

(5) Osteoporosis

(6) ± hyperglycemia

(7) ± hyperpigmentation

(8) Hypertension

(9) Thin skin

(10) Easy bruising

(11) Hirsutism

(12) Amenorrhea

(13) Depression

b. Laboratory

(1) Dexamethasone suppression test

↑ plasma cortisol

(2) 24-hour urine cortisol test

↑ urine cortisol

3. TREATMENT

Adrenal or pituitary surgery is the usual therapy indicated.

VI. OSTEOPOROSIS

A. DEFINITION

1. A metabolic bone disease characterized by an absolute ↓ in the amount of bone mass required for adequate mechanical support of the body.

2. The bones become ↑ fragile, then brittle and are predisposed to atraumatic fractures.

a. Vertebrae

b. Distal radius

c. Hip

3. Osteoporosis may be primary or secondary

4. Common etiologies

a. **Type I (Postmenopausal) Osteoporosis**

(1) Women ≈ 15-20 years postmenopause

(2) ↑ loss of trabecular bone

b. **Type II (Age-related or senile) Osteoporosis**

(1) Men and women >70 years of age

(2) A loss of both trabecular and cortical bone

B. DIAGNOSIS

1. History and Physical

a. **Usually asymptomatic until a fracture occurs**

b. Back pain

c. ↓ height

d. Dowager's hump (Kyphosis)

e. Fractures with minimal or no significant trauma

2. Laboratory
    a. Normal calcium and phosphorus
    b. Normal alkaline phosphatase
    c. X-rays
        (1) Early changes in the vertebra
            (a) Vertical striations of vertebral bodies
            (b) Relative accentuation of cortical plates
            (c) ↑ width of intervertebral spaces
        (2) Late changes in vertebra
            (a) Fractures
                ‣ Compression
                ‣ Crush
                ‣ Wedge
                ‣ Cortical plate
    d. DEXA (Dual-energy X-ray absorptiometry)
        Can detect a ↓ of 2% bone mass in clinical settings.

C. TREATMENT
    1. Exercise
    2. Calcium supplements
    3. Hormone replacement therapy
        a. Women
            Estrogen ± progesterone
        b. Men
            Testosterone if the serum level is low
    4. Calcitonin
    5. Vitamin D
        Reserved for patients with impaired calcium absorption.
    6. Biphosphonates
    7. Sodium fluoride

VII. **GOUT**
    A. DEFINITION
        1. A metabolic disease characterized by urate crystal deposition in the joints, subcutaneous tissues or kidneys.
        2. Classification
            a. Primary
                (1) Metabolic
                    (a) Idiopathic overproduction.............≈10% of cases
                    (b) Specific enzyme defects................. rare
                    (c) Renal idiopathic underexcretion......≈90% of cases

   b. Secondary

    (1) Metabolic

     (a) ↑ nucleic acid turnover

     (b) Glucose-6-phosphatase deficiency

    (2) Renal

     (a) Volume depletion

     (b) Chronic or acute renal failure

  3. Four clinical syndromes

   a. Asymptomatic hyperuricemia

   b. Acute gouty arthritis

   c. Chronic tophaceous gout

   d. Nephrolithiasis

B. DIAGNOSIS

  1. History and Physical

   a. Asymptomatic hyperuricemia

    ↑ plasma urate level >7.0 mg/dL

   b. Acute gouty arthritis

    (1) Monarticular pain (By frequency)

     (a) Great toe

      The first metatarsophalangeal joint (podagra)

     (b) Instep

     (c) Ankle

     (d) Heel

     (e) Knees

     (f) Wrist

     (g) Fingers

     (h) Elbows

    (2) ± fever

    (3) Later attacks are more severe and may be polyarticular

   c. Chronic tophaceous gout

    (1) A destructive arthropathy characterized by long standing deposition of monosodium urate around the joints and subcutaneous tissues.

    (2) Location

     (a) Antihelix of the ear

     (b) Extensor aspect of peripheral joints

   d. Nephrolithiasis

    (1) Acute urate nephropathy

     (a) Deposition of urate *within* the renal tubules

      Usually secondary to lympho- or myeloproliferative disorders or following chemotherapy.

             (2) Uric acid urolithiasis

    2. Laboratory

        a. Acute gouty arthritis

            (1) ↑ serum uric acid

            (2) ↑ sedimentation rate

            (3) CBC

                ± leukocytosis

            (4) Synovial fluid examination under a polarizing lens

                Needle-shaped, birefringent urate crystals *within* white blood cells

C. TREATMENT

    1. Acute gouty arthritis

        a. Decrease inflammation

            (1) NSAIDs

            (2) Colchicine

                If there is a contraindication to NSAIDs

            (3) Steroids

                (a) Intra-articular

                (b) Systemic

        b. Prophylaxis

            (1) Diet

                (a) **Low purine diet**

                (b) ↓ ETOH

        c. Weight loss

        d. Xanthine oxidase inhibitor

            Allopurinol

        e. ± uricosuric

            (1) Probenecid

            (2) Sulfinpyrazone

VII. **HYPERLIPOPROTEINEMIAS**

    A. DEFINITION

        1. **An ↑ of the *cholesterol* >200 mg/dL and/or**

        2. **An ↑ of the *triglycerides* >200 mg/dL**

        3. Cholesterol can be separated

            a. LDL

                Atherogenic lipoprotein

                    LDL <130 mg/dL

            c. HDL

                Antiatherogenic lipoprotein

                    HDL >35 mg/dL

4. **Primary hyperlipoproteinemia**

A *single gene mutation* which manifests a *primary* biochemical defect

5. Secondary hyperlipoproteinemia

    a. A systemic disease or drug which induces an↑ in plasma lipoproteins

        (1) Diabetes mellitus

        (2) Uremia

        (3) Systemic lupus erythematosus

        (4) Primary biliary cirrhosis

        (5) Extrahepatic biliary obstruction

        (6) Drug induced

            (a) Alcohol

            (b) Oral contraceptives

            (c) Glucocorticoids

B. DIAGNOSIS

1. Serum Lipoproteins

    a. Chylomicrons............................Triglycerides

    b. Very-low-density lipoproteins.....Triglycerides

    c. Low-density lipoproteins............Cholesterol

    d. High-density lipoproteins...........Cholesterol

2. Lipoprotein typing

    a. Type 1.....................................↑ chylomicrons

    b. Type 2a...................................↑ LDL (*Most common*)

    c. Type 2b...................................↑ LDL + VLDL

    d. Type 3.................................... ↑ chylomicron remnants + BetaVLDL

    e. Type 4.....................................↑ VLDL

    f. Type 5.....................................↑ VLDL + chylomicrons

3. *Hypercholesterolemia* (Type 2a)

    a. Mild hypercholesterolemia

        (1) Cholesterol......200-239 mg/dL

        (2) LDL................130-159 mg/dL

    b. Moderate hypercholesterolemia

        (1) Cholesterol......240-300 mg/dL

        (2) LDL................160-210 mg/dL

    c. Severe hypercholesterolemia

        (1) Cholesterol......>300 mg/dL

        (2) LDL................>210 mg/dL

4. *Hypertriglyceridemia*

    a. Moderate hypertriglyceridemia (Type 4)

        Triglycerides........250-500 mg/dL

b. Severe hypertriglyceridemia (Type 5)

Triglycerides.........>500 mg/dL

5. *Mixed Hyperlipidemias* (Types 2b, 3, 5)

C. TREATMENT

1. General
   a. **Low fat diet**
   b. Exercise
   c. Weight reduction if overweight
   d. Stop cigarette smoking
   e. ↓ ETOH
   f. If possible eliminate or control secondary causes

2. Hypercholesterolemia
   a. For moderate to severe disease
      (1) Bile acid sequestrants *and/or*
          Cholestyramine
      (2) Nicotinic acid *and/or*
      (3) HMG CoA Reductase Inhibitors
          (a) Lovastatin
          (b) Pravastatin
          (c) Simvastatin

3. Hypertriglyceridemia
   a. Moderate disease
      (1) Nicotinic acid
      (2) Fibric acid derivatives
          Gemfibrozil
   b. Severe disease
      (1) Very low fat diet (<10% calories as fat)
      (2) Fibric acid
          Gemfibrozil
      (3) **Triglyceride levels >1000 mg/dL can precipitate the development of acute pancreatitis.**

4. Mixed hyperlipidemias
   a. ↑ cholesterol + moderate ↑ triglycerides
      (1) HMG CoA Reductase Inhibitors
          (a) Lovastatin
          (b) Pravastatin
          (c) Simvastatin

I. **HEADACHES**
    A. Migraine or vascular headaches
        1. DEFINITION
            a. *Migraine with Aura* (Classic migraine headache)
                (1) DEFINITION
                    (a) A severe usually unilateral headache associated *with an aura* before onset and accompanied by neurologic, ophthalmologic, and gastro-intestinal signs and symptoms.
                    (b) It is a *recurrent headache* lasting a few hours to a couple of days
                    (c) A family history is common
                    (d) Women >60% of the cases
            b. *Migraine without aura* (Common migraine headache)
                (1) DEFINITION
                    (a) A severe, usually unilateral headache *not* associated with an aura before onset.
                    (b) *There are no neurologic signs and symptoms.*
                    (c) Common migraine is much more common than the classic migraine
                    (d) It is a *recurrent headache* lasting a few hours to three days
                    (e) A family history is common
                    (f) Women >60% of the cases
            c. Precipitating factors
                (1) "Body Stress"
                    (a) Fatigue
                    (b) Hunger
                    (c) Exhaustion
                    (d) Hypoglycemia
                    (e) ↑ emotional stress
                    (f) Menstruation
                    (g) Pregnancy
                (2) Diet
                    (a) Tyramine
                          ▸ Nuts
                          ▸ Cheese
                    (b) Nitrates
                        ▸ Smoked meats
                    (c) Phenylalanine
                    (d) Chocolate
                    (e) MSG
                    (f) ETOH

(3) Medications

Oral contraceptives

b. DIAGNOSIS

(1) History and Physical

(a) The Aura

- Onset about an hour *before* the headache and may continue past the onset of the headache.
- Ophthalmologic
  - Scotomas with scintillations
  - Visual field loss
- Unilateral paresthesias
- Hemiplegias
- Speech changes → aphasia
- Weakness
- Mood change

(b) The Headache

- **Headache**
  - Throbbing head pain
  - Usually unilateral
  - ↑ pain interferes with normal function
  - Movement and exercise↑ headache
- Nausea and vomiting
- Lightheadedness
- Diarrhea
- Vertigo
- Photophobia
- Phonophobia
- Chills

(2) Laboratory

Screening laboratory including CT of the head helps rule out secondary causes of headache.

c. TREATMENT

(1) Headache

(a) Sumatriptan

- IM
- Oral

(b) Analgesics

- Non-narcotic
- Narcotic

(c) Ergotamine

           (d) Antiemetics
- IM, oral, or suppository
  - Phenothiazine
  - Prochlorperazine
  - Promethazine

    (2) Prophylaxis

        (a) Avoid precipitating factors (Triggers)

        (b) Beta blockers

        (c) Calcium channel blockers

        (d) Antidepressants

3. *Cluster Headaches*

  a. DEFINITION

    (1) A very severe, unilateral headache which occurs in "clusters" of painful headaches through out the day lasting minutes to hours at a time, continuing on for weeks or months.

    (2) The headache-free period may last from months to years

    (3) Affects men ≈95% of the time

    (4) Precipitating factors

        (a) ETOH

        (b) Nicotine

        (c) ↑ stress

        (d) Vasodilators

  b. DIAGNOSIS

    (1) History and Physical

        (a) Headache
- **Excruciating, searing pain**
- Temporal, periorbital or orbital in location
- Onset is nocturnal

        (b) *Unilateral* Ophthalmologic findings
- Lacrimation
- Conjunctival congestion
- Miosis
- Ptosis
- Eyelid edema

        (c) Upper respiratory
- Nasal congestion
- Rhinorrhea

    (2) Laboratory

    Screening laboratory including CT of the head helps rule out secondary causes of headache.

c. TREATMENT

    (1) Oxygen at the time of a "cluster"

    (2) Sumatriptan

        (a) IM

        (b) Oral

    (3) Ergotamine

    (4) Antidepressants

    (5) Methysergide

        No more than 6 months (usual ≈3 months) at a time because of retroperitoneal or pleuropulmonary fibrosis

    (6) Calcium channel blockers

    (7) Prednisone

    (8) Lithium

    (9) Analgesics

        (a) Non-narcotic

        (b) Narcotic

B. *Tension (Muscle Contraction) Headaches*

  1. DEFINITION

    a. A headache characterized by a hatband tightening around the head.

    b. *Episodic tension headaches*

      The headache occurs during or after a stressful situation.

    c. *Chronic tension headaches*

      (1) A chronic headache which is present both day and night and is not responsive to OTC analgesics.

      (2) Psychological profiles of patients with chronic tension headaches reveal anxiety and depression.

  2. DIAGNOSIS

    a. History and Physical

      (1) The headache is

        (a) Generalized or bilateral

        (b) Bitemporal, suboccipital or fronto-occipital.

      (2) Movement doesn't increase the pain

      (3) Shoulders and upper backache

      (4) There is *no* nausea

      (5) The headache can last hours → days → months

    b. Laboratory

      Screening laboratory including CT of the head helps rule out secondary causes of headache

  3. TREATMENT

    a. Biofeedback

    b. Massage

    c. Psychotherapy

    d. Anxiolytics

    e. Antidepressants

    f. NSAIDs

    g Muscle relaxants

    h Analgesics

      (1) Non-narcotic

      (2) Narcotic (rarely indicated)

II. SEIZURES

  A. General

    1. **Seizure**

      A sudden alteration in consciousness associated with motor and/or sensory abnormalities produced by aberrant electrical discharge of cerebral neurons.

    2. **Epilepsy**

      Chronic or recurrent seizures

    3. Every patient that has a seizure is not an epileptic

    4. Every patient that has epilepsy has seizures

    5. Etiology of seizure

      a. Idiopathic.............≈75%

      b. Acquired..............≈25%

        (1) CNS infection

        (2) CNS tumor

        (3) Post-traumatic

        (4) Acute metabolic disease

        (5) Drug withdrawal

    6. Seizures may be generalized or partial

      a. Generalized seizures

        (1) The majority are characterized by at least some momentary loss of consciousness

        (2) The seizures may be convulsive or nonconvulsive

      b. Partial seizures

        (1) Simple

          (a) There is no alteration of consciousness

          (b) Usually originate from a focal structural lesion in the brain

          (c) May express a single symptom

        (2) Complex

          (a) There are *changing symptoms* associated with alteration in consciousness.

(b) Usually originate from a focal structural lesion in the brain

B. **Generalized convulsive seizures**

1. *Tonic-clonic (Grand Mal) Seizures*

a. DEFINITION

(1) Usually a 1-2 minute seizure characterized by a sudden loss of consciousness and

(a) Tonic contraction of the muscles

▸ A rigid (opisthotonic) posture

▸ Variable time frame usually in seconds but cyanosis can occur

(b) Clonic phase

▸ Jerky, rhythmic contractions of the muscles of all four extremities

▸ Urinary or fecal incontinence

▸ Trauma to the tongue secondary to biting

(c) Postictal phase

▸ A *gradual* return to consciousness

▸ Amnesia of the seizure

▸ Lethargy

▸ Muscle soreness

▸ Headache

b. DIAGNOSIS

(1) History and Physical

See above

(2) Laboratory

(a) Studies to rule out acquired forms of seizure disorders.

▸ CBC

▸ Chem 28

▸ Thyroid profile

▸ Drug screen

▸ Toxicology screen

▸ CT or MRI with *and* without contrast.

(b) EEG

▸ Interictal

• Normal ≈20% of the time

• Spike-slow complexes

• Bursts of abnormally slow activity

• Mixtures of spike and slow activity

▸ Ictal

•Tonic phase

○ Initial low-voltage fast (10 Hz or more) waves

○ Slow conversion to slower larger sharp waves in both hemispheres
- Clonic phase
    ○ Rapidly repeating spike discharges followed by sharp-slow activity
    ▸ Postictal
    Abnormally slow for hours after the seizure

c. TREATMENT
    (1) **Valproic acid**
    (2) Carbamazepine
    (3) Phenytoin
    (4) Phenobarbital

C. **Generalized nonconvulsive seizures**
    1. *Absence (Petit Mal) Seizures*
      a. DEFINITION
        (1) A seizure characterized by brief lapses of consciousness usually lasting 2-30 seconds.
        (2) **There is no convulsive activity or loss of postural control.**
        (3) They occur frequently and in severe cases can occur hundreds of times a day.
        (4) No structural lesion in the brain or metabolic disease has been identified
        (5) There is a genetic influence
        (6) They usually begin in childhood
      b. DIAGNOSIS
        (1) History and Physical
          (a) A blank stare as the seizure begins
          (b) ± *minor* motor activity
            ▸ Eyelid fluttering
            ▸ Upward rotation of the eyes
            ▸ Lip-smacking or chewing
            ▸ Slight twitching or shaking of the extremities
        (2) Laboratory
          (a) Studies to rule out acquired forms of seizure disorders.
            ▸ CBC
            ▸ Chem 28
            ▸ Thyroid profile
            ▸ Drug screen
            ▸ Toxicology screen
            ▸ CT or MRI with *and* without contrast.

(b) EEG

Repeated bursts and runs of 3.5-Hz spike-wave discharges

3. TREATMENT

    a. **Ethosuximide**

    b. **Valproic acid**

    c. Clonazepam

D. **Partial seizures**

    1. *Simple Partial Seizures*

        a. DEFINITION

            (1) A single or focal area of dysfunctional cerebral cortex produces abnormal electrical activity in the brain and a seizure occurs.

            (2) There is no alteration of consciousness.

            (3) **The characteristics of the seizure are dependent upon the location of the cortical lesion.**

                (a) *Partial motor seizures*

                    ▸ Clonic seizure movements of one part of the body

                        • Hands

                        • Face

                        • Fingers

                    ▸ Crude vocalizations or speech arrest

                    ▸ Dependent upon location a generalized seizure may occur

                (b) **Jacksonian seizures**

                    ▸ Primary motor (rolandic) seizures

                    ▸ The abnormal impulses spread to adjacent areas of the cortex hence, a rhythmic, clonic twitching of the thumb → hand →arm → face

                    ▸ A generalized seizure may occur

                    ▸ Todd's paralysis

                        A postictal paralysis of the limb affected by the seizure

                (c) *Partial sensory seizures*

                    ▸ Classic epileptic aura

                    ▸ Epileptiform discharges in contralateral sensory cortex

                        • Paresthesias

                        • Simple visual hallucinations

                        • Simple auditory hallucinations

                        • Vertigo

                    ▸ Temporal or frontal lobes

                        • Déjà vu

                        • Inappropriate anger or sadness

                        • Illusions

                      • Complex hallucinations

b. DIAGNOSIS
- (1) History and Physical
  - See above
- (2) Laboratory
  - (a) Studies to rule out acquired forms of seizure disorders.
    - ‣ CBC
    - ‣ Chem 28
    - ‣ Thyroid profile
    - ‣ Drug screen
    - ‣ Toxicology screen
    - ‣ CT or MRI with *and* without contrast.
  - (b) EEG
    - The electroencephalogram will identify abnormal patterns of brain activity in the affected cortical area.

c. TREATMENT
- (1) **Carbamazepine**
- (2) Phenytoin

2. *Complex partial (Psychomotor or Temporal lobe) Seizures*

a. DEFINITION
- (1) A single or "limited area" of dysfunctional *temporal lobe* cortex produces abnormal electrical activity in the brain and a seizure occurs. This abnormal activity *spreads* to extratemporal sites.
- (2) It is the most frequent form of chronic epilepsy
- (3) The structural lesions can be caused by
  - (a) Tumor
  - (b) Abscess
  - (c) Trauma
    - ‣ Birth injury
    - ‣ Postnatal trauma
  - (d) Infarction
- (4) The seizure is characterized by
  - (a) Aura
  - (b) Automatisms
    - ‣ Lip-smacking
    - ‣ Chewing
    - ‣ Walking in circles
    - ‣ Gesticulations
    - ‣ Complex automatisms
      - • Playing a complex piece of music

> > > > • Driving a car
> > > (c) Visual hallucinations
> > > (d) Auditory hallucinations
> > > (e) The seizure *can* become generalized with tonic-clonic activity and loss of consciousness
> > (5) Postictal state
> > > (a) Confusion
> > > (b) Headache
> > > (c) Exhaustion
> > > (d) Amnesia of events which occurred during the seizure
> > (6) ± abnormal interictal behavior
> > > (a) Circumstantiality
> > > (b) Self-absorption
> > > (c) Hypergraphia
> > > (d) Religiosity
> > > (e) Ruminative obsessiveness

> b. DIAGNOSIS
> > (1) History and Physical
> > > See above
> > (2) Laboratory
> > > (a) Studies to rule out acquired forms of seizure disorders.
> > > > ‣ CBC
> > > > ‣ Chem 28
> > > > ‣ Thyroid profile
> > > > ‣ Drug screen
> > > > ‣ Toxicology screen
> > > > ‣ CT or MRI with *and* without contrast.
> > (3) EEG
> > > (a) Temporal lobe spikes or slow foci
> > > (b) Surface EEG may be normal and abnormal activity may be recorded with sphenoidal or deep electrodes in the hippocampus or amygdala

> c. TREATMENT
> > (1) **Carbamazepine**
> > (2) Phenytoin
> > (3) Valproic acid

E. Febrile Seizures
> 1. DEFINITION
> > a. Characterized by a *generalized, nonfocal seizure* which occurs during the rapid rise of fever in a child with no history of CNS pathology.
> > b. Usually occurs between 6 months and 5 years

c. Fever ↓ seizure threshold
d. These children rarely develop epilepsy
2. TREATMENT
a. Oral or rectal acetaminophen
b. For seizures >15 minutes, diazepam via IV, IM or rectal suppository
c. ↑ risk children are placed on phenobarbital

III. INFECTION
A. *Bacterial Meningitis*
1. DEFINITION
a. A bacterial infection causing mild, moderate or severe inflammation of the pia-arachnoid and the cerebrospinal fluid which surrounds it.
b. *Acute bacterial meningitis is a medical emergency*
c. ↑ a favorable prognosis while ↓ the complications is a function of time between the onset of disease and beginning antibiotic therapy.
d. Etiologies
(1) Etiologies of ≈80% of cases
(a) *H influenzae*
(b) *N meningitidis*
(c) *S pneumoniae*
(2) **Neonate (0-4 weeks)**
(a) *Escherichia coli*
(b) *Streptococcus agalactiae*
(c) *Listeria monocytogenes*
(3) **Infant (1-3 months)**
(a) *Escherichia coli*
(b) *Streptococcus agalactiae*
(c) *Listeria monocytogenes*
(d) *Hemophilus influenzae*
(e) *Streptococcus pneumoniae*
(4) **Childhood/Adolescents (3 months-8 years)**
(a) *Hemophilus influenzae*
(b) *Streptococcus pneumoniae*
(c) *Neisseria meningitidis*
(5) **Adults (8-60 years)**
(a) *Streptococcus pneumoniae*
(b) *Neisseria meningitidis*
(6) **Adults (>60 years)**
(a) *Streptococcus pneumoniae*
(b) Gram-negative bacilli

(c) *Listeria monocytogenes*

2. DIAGNOSIS
    a. History and Physical
        (1) **Headache**
        (2) **Fever and chills**
        (3) **Meningismus**
        (4) Nausea and vomiting
        (5) Photophobia
        (6) ↑ diaphoresis
        (7) Weakness
        (8) Seizures
        (9) Focal neurologic deficits
        (10) Altered mental status
    b. Laboratory
        (1) **Lumbar puncture**
            (a) ↑ numbers of leukocytes, mostly neutrophils, in CSF
                Usually 1,000-10,000 cells/ml.
            (b) ↑ CSF pressure
                >180 mm of water
            (c) ↑ protein levels
                >150 mg/dL
            (d) ↓ sugar level
                <40 mg/dL
            (e) Gram stain
                + 80% of the time
            (f) CSF cultures
                + 70-80% of the time
        (2) Blood cultures
            + 40-60% of the time for *H influenzae, N meningitidis,* and *S pneumoniae*
        (3) CBC
            ↑ WBCs with a shift to the left
        (4) X-rays
            Studies to check for occult infection in the lungs, sinuses and skull

3. TREATMENT
    a. Minimum therapy is 10 days or seven days *after* becoming febrile
    b. Neonates
        (1) Ampicillin + a third-generation cephalosporin *or*
        (2) Ampicillin + an aminoglycoside

      c. Infants

          Ampicillin + a third-generation cephalosporin

      d. Children and Adolescents

          (1) Ampicillin + chloramphenicol

          (2) Third-generation cephalosporin

      e. Adults

          Third-generation cephalosporin

      f. Adults >50 years

          Ampicillin + a third-generation cephalosporin

4. PROGNOSIS

    a. Mortality

        (1) *H influenzae*............. $\approx$ 6%

        (2) *N meningitidis*.........$\approx$10%

        (3) *S pneumoniae*...........$\approx$19%

5. COMPLICATIONS

    a. **Waterhouse-Friderichsen syndrome**

        (1) Fulminant meningococcemia

            (a) Initial petechial rash $\rightarrow$ purpural rash with central necrosis

            (b) Septic shock

            (c) Hemorrhagic infarction of adrenals

            (d) If not diagnosed early it can be fatal

    b. Sensorineural hearing loss

    c. Learning deficits

    d. Seizures

    e. Cranial nerve palsies

    f. Obstructive hydrocephalus

    g. Brain infarction

B. *Brain Abscess*

  1. DEFINITION

    a. An illness characterized by the formation of an abscess *within* the brain parenchyma.

    b. Pathogenesis

        (1) Contiguous spread..$\approx$45%

            (a) Paranasal sinuses

            (b) Middle ear

            (c) Dental infection

        (2) Trauma...$\approx$5%

            (a) Post-op infections

            (b) Penetrating wounds

(3) Hematogenous...≈25%
     (a) Pulmonary...≈50%
     (b) Heart, bone, skin, teeth, abdomen, pelvis..........≈50%
(4) Unknown...≈30%

c. Location of abscess (by frequency)
    (1) **Frontal**
    (2) Parietal
    (3) Cerebellar
    (4) Occipital

d. Pathology
    (1) Cerebritis → liquefactive necrosis → capsule formation

e. Etiologies
    (1) Mixed infection 30-60% of the time
       (a) Aerobic bacteria ≈66% of the time
          ▸ *Streptococcal* spp....................50-70%
          ▸ *Staphylococcus aureus*............10-15%
             Usually following CNS trauma or surgery
          ▸ Gram-negative bacilli
             • *E coli*
             • *Proteus* sp.
             • *Klebsiella* sp.
             • *Pseudomonas* sp.
             • *Enterobacter* sp.
       (b) Anaerobic bacteria ≈33% of the time
          ▸ *Bacteroides* spp.
          ▸ *Fusobacterium* sp.
          ▸ Anaerobic streptococci
          ▸ *Clostridium* sp.
    (2) Immunocompromised patients
       (a) *Toxoplasma gondii*
       (b) Aerobic gram-negative bacteria
       (c) *Candida* sp.
       (d) *Aspergillus* sp.
       (e) *Nocardia asteroides*
       (f) *Mycobacterium* sp.
       (g) *Cryptococcus neoformans*
       (h) *L monocytogenes*
    (3) *H influenzae*, *N meningitidis*, and *S pneumoniae* rarely cause a brain
       abscess

2. DIAGNOSIS
    a. History and Physical
        (1) Signs and symptoms of ↑ intracranial mass
            (a) Headache
            (b) Fever
            (c) Nausea and vomiting
            (d) Confusion
            (e) Lethargy
            (f) Mass effect
                Papilledema
            (g) Nuchal rigidity
        (2) Focal brain dysfunction
            (a) Seizures
            (b) Cranial nerve palsy
                Ocular palsy
            (c) Hemiparesis
            (d) Changes in intellect and affect
    b. Laboratory
        (1) MRI and CT are the tests of choice to diagnose brain abscess.
        (2) MRI and CT are the tests of choice to follow the progress of therapy.
3. TREATMENT
    a. Surgery
        (1) Aspiration
        (2) Complete excision
    b. Antibiotic therapy
        (1) Begin empiric therapy based on likely etiology and pathogenesis, then confirm with cultures if possible.
        (2) **Ear/mastoids**
            (a) Etiologies
                ▸ *Streptococcal* spp.
                ▸ *Bacteroides* sp.
                ▸ Enterobacteriaceae
            (b) Treatment
                Penicillin + metronidazole + a third-generation cephalosporin.
        (3) **Paranasal sinuses**
            (a) Etiologies
                ▸ *Streptococcal* spp.
                ▸ Bacteroides
                ▸ *Hemophilus* spp.

(b) Treatment

Penicillin + metronidazole

(4) Trauma

(a) Etiologies

▸ *Staphylococcus* spp.

▸ *Streptococcus* spp.

▸ *Clostridium* spp.

(b) Treatment

Nafcillin + penicillin + metronidazole

c. Treatment usually lasts 4-6 weeks

4. PROGNOSIS

Mortality ≈10%.

IV. **NEOPLASIA**

A. DEFINITION

1. Benign or malignant neoplastic lesions can occur in the CNS.

2. Tumor origin

a. Primary CNS tumors.............................≈50%

b. Metastatic CNS tumors.........................≈50%

(1) Lung......................≈40%

(2) Breast...................≈20%

(3) Melanoma..............≈20%

(4) Colorectum............≈ 9%

(5) Miscellaneous.........≈11%

3. Location

a. Intracranial.........................≈90%

b. Within the spinal canal..........≈10%

4. Age

a. Childhood CNS tumors are cerebellar........≈70%

b. Adult CNS tumors are supratentorial.........≈90%

5. **Histologic typing of common *primary malignant* adult brain tumors**

a. *Glioblastoma multiforme*..≈40% of tumors

An astrocytoma grade 3 or 4. A highly malignant supratentorial tumor. Although radiation therapy and chemotherapy are used to treat it, the prognosis is poor with a mean survival of ≈1 year.

b. *Astrocytoma* (including anaplastic astrocytoma)............≈35% of tumors

A slow-growing low grade supratentorial tumor which can be cured with surgical resection depending upon location. Radiation therapy is used to treat tumors which have not been completely resected. The prognosis ranges from 2-8 years with a mean survival of 5 years

c. *Lymphoma*..≈10% of patients

Primary central nervous system lymphoma has been increasing in frequency. Occurs frequently in AIDS and immunosuppressed patients but may occur in immunocompetent individuals. The lesion is hyperintense on pre-gadolinium T1-weighted MRI. The tumor may be multifocal. Following biopsy and tissue diagnosis, glucocorticoids and chemotherapy is the treatment of choice. Radiation therapy is usually reserved for immunocompromised patients. The mean survival following therapy is 2 years.

d. *Oligodendroglioma*...≈5% of tumors

The majority of these tumors are low grade but highly anaplastic forms occur. It is a supratentorial tumor that usually presents in the frontal lobes. The tumor may have a benign or malignant histological appearance. Those tumors which have not been completely resected *or* those tumors with mixed glial cell population are more likely to recur. Surgical resection is followed by radiation and chemotherapy are used for tumors not completely resected. The prognosis is variable with a mean survival of 5 years.

e. *Medulloblastoma*...≈2% of tumors

The most common PNET tumor (Primitive neuroectodermal tumor). 25% of all *childhood* brain tumors. It is a tumor of the posterior fossa, usually a cerebellar tumor in both children and adults. Surgical resection + radiation therapy + chemotherapy yields a five-year mean survival of a 55%

6. **Histologic typing of common *primary benign* adult brain tumors**

a. *Meningioma*..≈80% of tumors

The majority of these tumors are benign, however, there are seven subtypes of which the malignant and angioblastic types are more likely to recur. The location of the tumor is critical to the prognosis. If the tumor can be completely resected a cure is likely. If not, a recurrence is likely. Radiation therapy is used in the treatment of tumors which have not been completely resected. The prognosis is highly variable, but usually long term.

b. *Acoustic neuroma*...≈10% of tumors

These benign tumors also called an acoustic schwannoma can present with unilateral tinnitus and deafness. It is cured with surgery or focal irradiation with radiosurgery.

7. **Histologic typing of common *primary* childhood brain tumors**

a. Astrocytoma...........................≈30% of tumors

b. Brainstem gliomas...................≈20% of tumors

c. Medulloblastoma.....................≈20% of tumors

d. Ependymoma..........................≈ 9% of tumors

e. Craniopharyngioma.................≈ 3% of tumors

B. DIAGNOSIS
   1. History and Physical
      a. Signs and symptoms of ↑ intracranial mass
         (1) Headache
         (2) Nausea and vomiting
         (3) Confusion
         (4) Lethargy
         (5) Mass effect
            (a) Papilledema
            (b) Herniation
      b. Focal brain dysfunction
         (1) Seizures
         (2) Cranial nerve palsy
         (3) Hemiparesis
         (4) Changes in intellect and affect
   2. Laboratory
      a. MRI is superior to CT scan for the diagnosis of brain tumor.
      b. Myelography is helpful in diagnosing posterior fossa tumors.
      c. Angiography is used pre-op to delineate the size and blood flow of the tumor.
      d. Lumbar puncture for cytologic evaluation of malignant cells.
         (1) **Do not perform a lumbar puncture (because of possible herniation) if:**
            (a) Unexplained papilledema
            (b) A suspected mass lesion in the brain
   3. TREATMENT AND PROGNOSIS
      See above

V. **STROKE**
   A. GENERAL
      1. *Transient Ischemic Attack* (TIA)
         The abrupt onset of a focal neurological defect resulting from ischemia that *fully resolves* within 24 hours.
      2. *Reversible ischemic neurologic deficit*
         The abrupt onset of a focal neurological defect resulting from ischemia that lasts longer than 24 hours but *fully resolves* in less than a week.
      3. *Stroke*
         a. The abrupt onset of a focal neurological deficit secondary to pathology involving the intracranial or extracranial blood vessels.
            (1) Progressing stroke (stroke in evolution)
               Neurologic changes are in evolution, unstable and progressive

(2) Completed stroke

Neurologic changes are stable and nonprogressive

4. Major risk factors in stroke

    a. Cardiovascular

        (1) Hypertension

        (2) Congestive heart failure

        (3) MI

        (4) Atrial fibrillation

    b. Metabolic

        (1) Hyperlipidemia

        (2) Diabetes mellitus

    c. Habituations

        (1) Smoking

        (2) Acute alcohol abuse

5. Classification

    a. Ischemic stroke..........................≈80% of cases

    b. Hemorrhagic stroke...................≈20% of cases

B. *Ischemic stroke*

1. DEFINITION

    a. There is inadequate perfusion of the brain parenchyma secondary to obstruction of the blood vessel resulting in tissue necrosis.

    b. Depending on the cerebrovascular pathology the injury may be focal, multifocal or diffuse.

    c. The obstruction of the blood vessel may be caused by thrombus formation, embolism or vasoconstriction

    d. Common etiologies contributing to stroke

        (1) Atherosclerosis

        (2) Embolization

            (a) Heart disease

                ▸ Valvular

                ▸ Atrial fibrillation

                ▸ Mural thrombus

        (3) Vasculitides

        (4) Hematologic disorders

            (a) Platelet disorders

                ▸ Thrombocytosis >600,000/mm^3

                ▸ Platelet hyperaggregability

            (b) Hematocrit >55 mL/dL

            (c) WBC >500,000 cells/mm^3

        (5) Hemoglobinopathies

(6) Autoimmunopathies
    (a) Sickle cell disease
    (b) Lupus anticoagulant
(7) Drug induced
    (a) Oral contraceptives
    (b) ETOH
    (c) "Street Drugs"
        ‣ Cocaine
        ‣ Amphetamines
  e. **Cerebral embolism is the most common cause of ischemic stroke.**

2. DIAGNOSIS
  a. History and Physical
    (1) Ischemic (Thromboembolic) stroke presents with *no warning*.
    (2) There is sudden onset associated with a maximal neurologic deficit.
    (3) The clinical findings are dependent upon the size and the distribution of the vessel involved.
  b. Laboratory
    (1) Diagnosis of diseases which predispose to stroke
      (a) CBC
      (b) Chem 28
      (c) PT/PTT
      (d) Sedimentation rate
      (e) RPR
      (f) ECG
      (g) Chest X-ray
    (2) Special studies if history or screening laboratory is abnormal
      (a) Transthoracic echocardiogram
      (b) Screening for hypercoaguable states
    (3) Screening of carotid artery and other vessels for disease
      (a) Carotid ultrasound or Doppler examination
      (b) Magnetic resonance angiography is superior to
    (4) MRI is superior to CT for diagnosis of *ischemic stroke*.
    (5) Selective cerebral arteriography is used in special cases.

3. TREATMENT
  a. Anticoagulation
  b. Antiplatelet agents
  c. Surgical endarterectomy
  d. Reduce risk factors
    (1) Stop smoking
    (2) Normalize blood pressure slowly

(3) Aspirin or ticloidine daily

(4) Maintain good control of diabetes mellitus

(5) Moderate the use of alcohol

e. Corticosteroids are contraindicated in the treatment of stroke

4. PROGNOSIS

    a. Acute completed stroke during hospitalization

        Mortality............................≈25%

    b. Good functional recovery.........≈40%

F. *Hemorrhagic stroke*

    1. GENERAL

        a. Intracranial hemorrhage...........................≈20% of all strokes

            (1) Subarachnoid space.............≈50% of the time

            (2) Intracerebral.......................≈50% of the time

    2. *Subarachnoid hemorrhage*

        a. DEFINITION

            (1) A stoke characterized by the hemorrhage of blood over the surface of the brain.

            (2) Etiologies

                (a) Head trauma

                (b) Rupture of a blood vessel

                (c) Arterial aneurysm

                    ▸ **Saccular (Berry) aneurysm**

                        Accounts for ≈80% of cases

                    ▸ Fusiform aneurysm

                        Secondary to atherosclerosis

                    ▸ Mycotic aneurysm

                        Secondary to septic emboli

                (d) Vascular malformation

                (e) Blood dyscrasia

                (f) "Drug abuse"

                    ▸ Cocaine

                    ▸ Amphetamine

                (g) Tumor

        b. DIAGNOSIS

            (1) History and Physical

                (a) The clinical findings are dependent upon the size and the distribution of the vessel involved.

                (b) *Anatomic changes* that can occur *before* the aneurysmal rupture

                    ▸ Sentinel leaks

                    ▸ Compression of surrounding tissues

> ‣ Embolization of aneurysmal clot

(c) *Prodromal signs and symptoms* of arterial aneurysms

> ‣ Headache
> ‣ Nausea and vomiting
> ‣ Neck stiffness

(d) *Rupture of the aneurysm*

> ‣ Loss of consciousness ≈50% of the time
> ‣ Meningeal irritation
> ‣ Neck stiffness
> ‣ Photophobia
> ‣ ↑ blood pressure
> ‣ Focal neurologic deficits
> ‣ Seizures
> ‣ Retinal hemorrhage
> ‣ Fever
> ‣ Leukocytosis

(e) *Late changes*

> ‣ Delirium
> ‣ ± diffuse mild upper motor abnormalities
>   May indicate development of communicating hydrocephalus
> ‣ Inappropriate ↑ of ADH
>   Hyponatremia

(2) Laboratory

(a) CT is superior to MRI for the detection of subarachnoid hemorrhage

(b) If the CT is *nondiagnostic*, perform a lumbar puncture
    Check for blood or xanthochromia

(c) Cerebral angiography is the definitive study to detect the source of a subarachnoid hemorrhage.

c. TREATMENT

(1) Strict bed rest

(2) Analgesics
    Nonopiate

(3) Nimodipine
    A calcium channel blocker that ↓ incidence of cerebral infarction by ≈33% of the time

(4) Neurologically stable

(a) Surgery
    Clipping the aneurysm to prevent further hemorrhage

d. PROGNOSIS
  (1) Mortality is ≈66% at one month
  (2) Of the survivors ≈25% are severely disabled
3. *Intracerebral hemorrhage*
  a. DEFINITION
    a. A nontraumatic spontaneous hemorrhage that occurs primarily within the brain parenchyma or intracerebral tissues.
    b. Etiologies
      (1) "Hypertensive" atherosclerotic hemorrhage
        (a) ≈60% occur in hypertensives
        (b) Usually catastrophic
        (c) Derives from degenerative-atherosclerotic vascular injury
      (2) Lobar
        (a) More common in elderly
          ‣ Associated with amyloid angiopathy
        (b) In younger patients
          ‣ Small vascular malformations
          ‣ Sympathomimetic drug abuse
        (c) Not always catastrophic
      (3) Vascular malformation
  b. DIAGNOSIS
    (1) General
      (a) Severe headache
      (b) Nausea and vomiting
      (c) Loss of consciousness
      (d) Severe hypertension
      (e) ± seizures
    (2) *Location* of the "hypertensive" hemorrhage within the brain parenchyma
      (a) Basal ganglia-internal capsule..........................≈40%
        ‣ Severe headache ipsilateral to bleed
        ‣ Coma
        ‣ Seizures
        ‣ Contralateral hemiplegia
        ‣ Eyes deviate toward lesion
      (b) Lobar
        ‣ Peripheral lesions in the white matter ......≈22%
          • Cerebrum or cerebellum
        ‣ Usually less severe
        ‣ Fewer acute or permanent neurologic abnormalities
        ‣ Signs and symptoms dependent upon location

           (c) Thalamus..≈15%
- Moderate headache, unilateral or global
- Drowsiness → coma
- Contralateral hemiparesis
- Hemianopsia
- Deviation of eyes down and contralateral to lesion

           (d) Pontine..≈8%
- Severe global headache
- ↑ lethargy or coma
- Bilateral conjugate gaze paralysis or ocular bobbing
- Pinpoint pupils
- Stertorous or irregular bleeding
- Decerebrate or decorticate rigidity

           (e) Cerebellar..≈8%
- Moderate → severe occipital headache
- Stupor → coma with brain stem compression
- dysarthria
- Ipsilateral incoordination-ataxia
- Facial weakness
- Paralysis of ipsilateral conjugate gaze

      (3) Laboratory
           (a) CT will demonstrate the area(s) of hemorrhage but not etiology
           (b) If the bleed is not catastrophic
              ± arteriography for potentially treatable lesion
           (c) Avoid lumbar puncture because it may precipitate intracranial herniation

c. TREATMENT
      (1) Medical
           (a) Guard against herniation
- Glucocorticoids
- Osmotic agents
- Diuretics

           (b) Control the blood pressure
- **Do not drop the blood pressure precipitously**
              Lower the blood pressure slowly over days

           (c) Control any bleeding diathesis
      (2) Surgical
           (a) Evacuation of the clot
               Brain stem or cerebellar bleed

(b) Correction of arteriovenous malformation or aneurysm

(c) Ventricular drainage or shunt

d. PROGNOSIS

(1) Most patients in coma do not survive

(2) Prognosis is best for hemorrhage in the peripheral cerebral or cerebellar hemispheres.

VI. PARKINSON'S DISEASE

A. DEFINITION

1. It is one of the akinetic rigid syndromes characterized by

a. Resting tremor

b. Cogwheel rigidity

c. Bradykinesia

d. Akinesis

e. Impaired postural reflexes

2. Most common age that symptoms begin is 60 years

3. Etiology is unknown

a. Drug-induced parkinsonism

(1) Phenothiazines

(2) Butyrophenones

b. Postencephalitic parkinsonism

Following the 1918-1926 pandemic of lethargic encephalitis

4. Pathology

Degeneration of the pigmented, dopamine-containing neurons of the pars compacta of the substantia nigra

B. DIAGNOSIS

1. Early disease is usually confined to a limb or a hemiparetic distribution

a. ± weakness

b. Tremor

c. Fatigue

d. Muscle slowness or stiffness

2. As the disease progresses

a. Simian posture

(1) Stiff forward stoop with bent knees, hips and neck

(2) Arms held close to the body and flexed at the elbow

b. Gait

(1) Small and shuffling

(2) Late disease

(a) Festination

▸ Uncontrolled acceleration of their gait

(b) Retropulsion
c. Trembling hands with pill rolling posture
d. Masked face
e. ↓ spontaneous blinking
    (1) Myerson's sign
        Failure of blink reflex when the eyebrow is tapped
f. Altered handwriting
g. Cogwheel rigidity of the extremities
    Nonspastic, steadily ↑ resistance to movement, often interrupted by tremor
h. Psychiatric
    (1) The majority of patients develop depression
    (2) Dementia in ≈50% of patients by seven or more years

C. TREATMENT
  1. Medical
    a. Selegiline
    b. Anticholinergics
      (1) Trihexyphenidyl
      (2) Benztropine
      (3) Amantadine
    c. Dopamine agonists
      (1) Bromocriptine
      (2) Pergolide
    d. Caridopa/levodopa
      (1) After 5-7 years 25-50% maintain their initial improvement
        (a) Peak-dose dyskinesias
        (b) Wearing-off phenomenon
  2. Surgical
    a. Experimental therapies
      (1) Stereotaxic thalamotomy
      (2) Stereotaxic pallidotomy
      (3) Transplantation of dopamine-generating fetal cells

VII. **ALZHEIMER'S DISEASE**
  A. DEFINITION
    1. Alzheimer's disease is a degenerative dementia characterized by the loss of function in *multiple* cognitive abilities.
      a. Classically, it was described as a *presenile dementia*
        Presenting in late middle life but *preceding* the senile period
      b. The identical illness occurs in very old patients and is named
        Senile dementia of the Alzheimer's type

2. It is the most frequently diagnosed dementia in North America
3. Etiology is unknown
4. **There is a loss of memory and other cognitive functions over time.**
5. Pathology
    a. Death and disappearance of nerve cells in the cerebral cortex
    b. Microscopic
        (1) Neurofibrillary tangles
        (2) Neuritic plaques

B. DIAGNOSIS
    1. History and physical
        a. Initial stage
            (1) Loss of short-term memory
            (2) Language deficits
                (a) Speech content
                (b) Comprehension
                (c) Naming
                (d) Verbal fluency
            (3) Visuospatial dysfunction
                (a) Spatial dyscoordination
                (b) Object recognition
                (c) Distance estimation
            (4) Inability to execute executive functions
                (a) Problem solving
                (b) Concept formation
                (c) Planning
        b. Middle stage
            (1) Behavioral symptoms
                (a) Agitation
                (b) Depression
                (c) Anxiety
                (d) Wandering
                (e) Insomnia
                (f) Delusions
                (g) Hallucinations
        c. Late stage
            (1) Extrapyramidal signs
                (a) Shuffling, short steps
                (b) Generalized muscle stiffness
                (c) Myoclonus
            (2) Seizures

        d. Terminal

            Nearly decorticate in a state of total helplessness

    2. Mental status testing

        a. Blessed Information-Memory-Concentration test

        b. Mini Mental State Examination

    3. Laboratory

        a. Rule out underlying causes of dementia

            (1) CBC

            (2) Chem-28

            (3) Thyroid profile

            (4) Urinalysis

            (5) RPR

            (6) ECG

            (7) Chest X-ray

            (8) Vitamin B_{12} and folate levels

            (9) CT or MRI

C. TREATMENT

    1. Behavioral symptoms

        a. Anxiety

            (1) Benzodiazapines

            (2) Low-dose neuroleptics

        b. Depression

            (1) Tricyclic antidepressants

            (2) Serotonin re-uptake inhibitors

        c. Agitation and/or psychotic symptoms

            Neuroleptics

        d. Cognitive symptoms

            Tacrine

                A long-acting, reversible cholinesterase inhibitor

I. RED BLOOD CELL DISORDERS
    A. Myeloproliferative disorders
        1. *Polycythemia vera*
            a. DEFINITION
                (1) A neoplastic disease of the bone marrow stem cell which is characterized by an uncontrolled expansion of all bone marrow elements with an ↑ in erythroid series predominating.
                (2) The etiology is unknown
                (3) There is an increase in the red blood cell mass
                (4) **Relative polycythemia**
                    (a) Normal red cell mass and a contracted plasma volume
                    (b) Usually occurs in obese, hypertensive males
                    (c) Hematocrit between 55-60%
                    (d) Aggressive phlebotomy is not indicated
            b. DIAGNOSIS
                (1) Signs and symptoms
                    (a) Headache
                    (b) Pruritus
                    (c) Plethora
                    (d) Tinnitus
                    (e) Dizziness
                    (f) Splenomegaly is usually present
                    (g) ± Hepatomegaly
                (2) Laboratory
                    (a) CBC
                        ▸ Leukocytosis
                        ▸ Basophilia
                        ▸ Thrombocytosis
                        ▸ Hematocrit >60%
                    (b) Bone marrow biopsy
                        ▸ Not diagnostic
                            • Panhyperplasia
                            • Slightly ↑ megakaryocyte
                  $(c)^{51}Cr$-labeled red cell mass
                        ▸ Differentiates between absolute and relative polycythemia

(3) Criteria for diagnosis

    (a) Three criteria from A *or* two criteria from A and two from B.

        ‣ Criteria A

            • ↑ Red cell mass

                ○ Males ≥36 ml/kg

                ○ Females ≥32 ml/kg

            • Normal arterial oxygen saturation ≥92%

            • Splenomegaly

        ‣ Criteria B

            • Thrombocytosis

                Platelets >400,000/μL

            • Leukocytosis

                ○ WBCs ≥12,000/μL

                ○ There must be an absence of infection

            • ↑ NAP score >

                ○ NAP >100

                ○ There must be an absence of infection or fever

            • ↑ B_{12} or UBBC

                ○ B_{12} >900 pg/ml

                ○ UBBC >2200 pg/ml

c. TREATMENT

    (1) Avoid over treatment

    (2) Control blood volume

        Phlebotomy to ↓ the hematocrit to 42-47%

    (3) Control of panmyelosis

        (a) <50 years of age

            Avoid myelosuppressive agents

        (b) Hydroxyurea

        (c) Phosphorus radiotherapy

            ‣ ↓ risk of thrombosis

            ‣ ↑ risk of leukemia, lymphoma and skin cancer

        (d) Chemotherapy

d. COMPLICATIONS

    (1) Intravascular hyperviscosity + abnormal platelets

        (a) MI

        (b) Venous thromboembolism

        (c) Stroke

e. PROGNOSIS

    Mean survival ≈10-12 years following diagnosis

B. *Anemia*

  1. DEFINITION

    a. A decrease in the hemoglobin content or red blood cell mass that is set below the physiologic threshold of oxygen demand of the tissues.

      (1) Adult males

        (a) Hemoglobin..............<14 g/dL *or*

        (b) Hematocrit................<41%

      (2) Adult females

        (a) Hemoglobin..............<12 g/dL *or*

        (b) Hematocrit................<36%

  2. *Iron deficiency anemia*

    a. DEFINITION

      (1) A hypochromic microcytic anemia

      (2) Etiologies

        (a) Blood loss

          ▸ Occult malignancy

          ▸ Menstrual

        (b) ↑ iron requirements

          ▸ Pregnancy

          ▸ Lactation

          ▸ Infancy

        (c) ↓ iron absorption

          ▸ Postgastrectomy

          ▸ Celiac disease

          ▸ Inflammatory bowel disease

        (d) Plummer-Vinson syndrome

          ▸ Esophageal webs

          ▸ Dysphagia

          ▸ Glossitis

    b. DIAGNOSIS

      (1) No early signs and symptoms

      (2) Late signs and symptoms

        (a) Fatigue

        (b) Headache

        (c) Dizziness

        (d) Shortness of breath

        (e) Exercise intolerance

        (f) Irritability

(3) Laboratory

    (a) CBC

        ‣ ↓ MCV

        ‣ ↓ MCHC

    (b) Peripheral smear

        ‣ Hypochromia

        ‣ Microcytic cells

        ‣ Anisocytosis

            • Different *sizes* of red blood cells

        ‣ Poikilocytosis

            • Different *shapes* of red blood cells

    (c) ↓ serum iron

        <60 μg/dL

    (d) ↑ total iron-binding capacity

        >360 μg/dL

    (e) ↓ serum ferritin

        <12 μg/L

    (f) ↑ serum transferrin receptor concentration

        >8.5 mg/L

c. TREATMENT

    (1) Identify the underlying etiology and correct it, if possible

    (2) Oral iron therapy

        (a) Ferrous sulfate

        (b) Ferrous gluconate

        (c) Ferrous fumarate

    (3) Parenteral iron therapy

        (a) Iron dextran

            ‣ Reserved for patients with

                • Intolerance of oral iron

                • Poor absorption

                • Massive or continuous blood loss

    (4) Monitor the patient

        (a) CBC and indices

        (b) Reticulocyte count

        (c) Serum ferritin

3. *Hemolytic anemia*

    a. DEFINITION

        (1) An anemia characterized by an ↑ rate of red blood cell destruction

        (2) Life span of RBCs

            (a) Normal............................90-120 days

(b) Moderate hemolysis............20-40 days
(c) Severe hemolysis.................5-20 days
(3) Etiologies
    (a) Intracorpuscular disorders
        ▸ Membrane defects
            Hereditary spherocytosis
            Hereditary elliptocytosis
        ▸ Enzyme defects
            G6PD deficiency
        ▸ Abnormal hemoglobin
            Sickle cell disease
        ▸ Abnormal synthesis of globulin
            Thalassemias
        ▸ Paroxysmal nocturnal hemoglobinuria
    (b) Extracorpuscular disorders
        ▸ Mechanical damage to RBCs
            • Severe aortic and mitral valve disease
            • Prosthetic valves
            • Microangiopathic hemolytic anemia
                ○ DIC
                ○ Thrombotic thrombocytopenic purpura
                ○ Malignant hypertension
                ○ Eclampsia
                ○ Giant hemangiomas
        ▸ Chemicals, toxins or infection
            • Heavy metals
            • Snake venom
            • Malaria
        ▸ Hypersplenism
            • Chronic hemolytic anemia of any etiology
            • Chronic infection
            • Malignancies
            • Rheumatoid arthritis
                ○ Felty's syndrome
        ▸ Antibody-induced
            • Cold-antibody
                ○ Idiopathic
                ○ Infection
                    · *Mycoplasma pneumoniae*
                    · Infectious mononucleosis

          ∘ Malignancy

            · Lymphoma

        • Warm-antibody

          ∘ Idiopathic

          ∘ Malignancy

            · Lymphoma

            · Leukemia

          ∘ Collagen-vascular diseases

          ∘ Drug-induced

b. DIAGNOSIS

    (1) History and Physical

        (a) A careful history

            Scrutiny concerning onset

    (2) Laboratory

        (a) CBC

            Mild → severe anemia

        (b) Peripheral smear

           ▸ Reticulocytosis

           ▸ Intracorpuscular

              • Spherocytes

                ∘ Hereditary spherocytosis

                ∘ Antibody-induced hemolytic anemia

              • Sickle cells

                Sickle cell disease and syndromes

              • Heinz bodies

                Thalassemias

              • Target cells

                Hemoglobin disorders

              • Basophilic stippling

                Lead poisoning

           ▸ Extracorpuscular

              • Schistocyte

                Mechanical damage to RBCs

              • Agglutinated cells

                Cold-agglutinin disease

        (c) Chem-28

           ▸ ↑ indirect bilirubin

           ▸ ↑ LDH

        (d) ↑ plasma hemoglobin

        (e) ↓ haptoglobin

(f) Urine
- ± hemosiderin
- ± hemoglobin

(g) Osmotic fragility test

↑ fragility of red blood cells in membrane disorders

(h) Ham test

+ in paroxysmal nocturnal hemoglobinuria

(i) Coombs' test

+ Warm-antibody hemolytic anemia

(j) Cold agglutinin titers

↑ in chronic cold agglutinin disease

c. TREATMENT

(1) Nonimmune hemolytic anemia

(a) Correction, if possible, of the underlying illness

(b) ± transfusion

(c) Splenectomy

(d) Corticosteroids

Paroxysmal nocturnal hemoglobinuria

(2) Antibody-induced hemolytic anemia

(a) ± transfusion

(b) Splenectomy

(c) Corticosteroids

(d) Immunosuppression
- Azathioprine
- Cyclophosphamide

(3) Drug-induced

Discontinuation of medication

4. *Aplastic anemia*

a. DEFINITION

(1) **Injury or destruction of the pluripotential stem cell.**

(2) Etiologies of *acquired* aplastic anemia

(a) **Idiopathic**

(b) Direct toxicity to the bone marrow
- Acute radiation
- Chemotherapeutics
- Benzene

(c) Idiosyncratic relationships
- Medications
  - Antibiotics
    - Chloramphenicol

                 ◦ Sulfas
- NSAIDs
- Antimalarials
    ▸ Organic compounds
- Insecticides
- Pesticides

(d) Paroxysmal nocturnal hemoglobinuria

(e) Infections may cause aplastic anemia but they are rare
    ▸ HIV
    ▸ Hepatitis non-A, non-B, non-C
    ▸ Infectious mononucleosis

b. DIAGNOSIS

  (1) History and physical

    (a) **Bleeding is the most common early symptom.**
      ▸ Petechiae
      ▸ Ecchymoses

    (b) Signs and symptoms of anemia
      ▸ Fatigue
      ▸ Dizziness
      ▸ Shortness of breath

  (2) Laboratory

    (a) CBC
      ▸ Moderate → severe anemia
      ▸ Neutropenia
      ▸ ↓ reticulocyte count
      ▸ Thrombocytopenia

    (b) Peripheral smear
      Pancytopenia

    (c) Bone marrow biopsy
      ▸ Pancytopenia
      ▸ Bone marrow with fatty replacement

c. TREATMENT

  (1) Attempt to alleviate any underlying etiology

  (2) ± transfusion

    (a) Red blood cells

    (b) Platelets

  (3) Watch for infection

  (4) Bone marrow transplant

  (5) Immunosuppression

    (a) Antithymocyte globulin therapy

    (b) Glucocorticoids

    (c) Cyclosporine

    (d) Growth factors

  d. PROGNOSIS

    The > the neutropenia and thrombocytopenia, the > the ↓ in survival

5. *Cobalamin deficiency anemia*

  a. DEFINITION

    (1) *A normochromic macrocytic anemia* caused by a deficiency of vitamin B_{12} or folic acid

    (2) Etiologies of megaloblastic anemias

      (a) Folic acid deficiency

        ► ↓ ingestion

          • Inadequate diet

          • ETOH

        ► ↓ absorption

          • Chronic intestinal disease

        ► Drugs

          • Folic acid antagonists

            ○ ETOH

            ○ Methotrexate

            ○ Trimethoprim

            ○ Oral contraceptives

            ○ Sulfasalazine

            ○ Anticonvulsants

        ► ↑ body need

          • Pregnancy

          • Chronic hemolysis

          • Malignancy

      (b) Vitamin B_{12} deficiency

        ► *Pernicious anemia*

          • ↓ intrinsic factor

            ○ **Gastric mucosal defect**

              · Atrophic gastritis

              · Histamine-fast achlorhydria

         • Intrinsic factor must be present for vitamin B_{12} to be absorbed in the terminal ileum.

         • The patient may develop *neurologic and/or psychiatric symptoms*.

           Combined systems disease

                 ▸ Gastrectomy
                 ▸ Ileitis or ileal resection
                 ▸ Parasites
                     Fish-tapeworm
                 ▸ GI bacterial overgrowth
                 ▸ Pancreatic insufficiency

b. DIAGNOSIS

   (1) History and physical

      (a) Fatigue and weakness

      (b) Glossitis

      (c) Weight loss

   (2) Laboratory

      (a) CBC

          ▸ Mild → moderate anemia

          ▸ MCV >94 fL.

          ▸ ± leukopenia

          ▸ ± thrombocytopenia

      (b) Peripheral smear

          ▸ Neutrophil hypersegmentation

          ▸ Anisocytosis

          ▸ Poikilocytosis

          ▸ Macro-ovalocytosis

      (c) ↓ serum cobalamin level

      (d) ↓ serum folate level

      (e) + Shilling test

      (f) ± serum antibodies to IF

c. TREATMENT

   (1) Identify underlying etiology and attempt to correct it

   (2) Folic acid deficiency

      (a) 1 mg of folic acid PO daily for 2-4weeks until normal diet is
          established.

      (b) With underlying chronic disease, continue indefinitely

   (2) Vitamin B_{12} deficiency

      1 mg IM daily for 1 week, then weekly x 8 weeks followed by 1 mg
      IM once a month for life

C. *Thalassemia*s

   1. DEFINITION

   A heterogeneous group of inherited disorders characterized by the ↓ synthesis of
   either the alpha- or beta-globin chains of the hemoglobin molecule.

2. DIAGNOSIS
    a. **α-Thalassemia**
        (1) No alpha-globulin genes present
            (a) *Homozygous α-thalassemia*
                ‣ Hydrops fetalis
                ‣ Death
        (2) One alpha-globulin gene present
            (a) *Hemoglobin H disease*
                ‣ Hypochromic, microcytic anemia
                ‣ Hemoglobin ≈7-10 gm/dL
                ‣ Heinz bodies
                ‣ Monitor for↑ anemia
                    • ± splenomegaly
                    • ± aplastic crisis
        (3) Two alpha-globulin genes present
            (a) *Heterozygous α-thalassemia-1* and *Homozygous α-thalassemia-2*
                ‣ α-thalassemia trait
                ‣ No anemia
                ‣ Peripheral smear
                ‣Microcytic hypochromic
        (4) Three alpha-globulin genes present
            (a) *Heterozygous α-thalassemia-3*
                ‣ Silent carrier
    b. **β-Thalassemia**
        (1) Multiple genetic mutations of the beta-globulin gene can result in multiple syndromes
        (2) Thalassemia major
            (a) *Homozygous β-thalassemia*
            (b) A childhood illness characterized by a severe hemolytic anemia.
            (c) Growth abnormalities
                ‣ ↑ in ineffective erythropoiesis causes profound↑ of the marrow space and distortion of bones.
                ‣ ↑ extramedullary hematopoiesis
            (d) Iron overload
                ‣ Causes tissue fibrosis affecting multiple organs
            (e) Hemoglobin 3-6 gm/dL
                ‣ Hemoglobin F is the major hemoglobin
                ‣ Hemoglobin A ↓ or absent, 2-5% hemoglobin A_2
            (f) Patients are dependent upon blood transfusion to sustain life

(3) Thalassemia intermedia
  (a) Double heterozygous for two *different* thalassemic mutations
  (b) Genetically variable
  (c) Hemoglobin 8-10 gm/dL
  (d) Similar to thalassemia major but with slower time course
  (e) Life expectancy to mid-adulthood
(4) Thalassemia minor
  (a) *Heterozygous β-thalassemia*
  (b) ± Mild anemia and changes in the peripheral smear.
    ‣ Anisocytosis
    ‣ Poikilocytosis
    ‣ Target cells
  (c) Hemoglobin 10-12 gm/dL
    ‣ Hemoglobin A is the major hemoglobin
    ‣ Hemoglobin A_2 and F ≈2-10%
  (d) Morbidity is not associated with this illness

3. TREATMENT
  a. **Thalassemias do not respond to iron therapy**
  b. Heterozygous α- and β-thalassemia
      Usually no therapy is indicated
  c. Transfusion to keep hemoglobin ≥8 gm/dL
  d. Splenectomy to ↓ hemolysis
  e. ± iron chelation therapy
      ↓ organ fibrosis

D. Hemoglobinopathies
  1. *Sickle cell Disease*
    a. DEFINITION
      (1) A group of inherited disorders that are characterized by structurally abnormal hemoglobin molecules that polymerize under ↓ oxygen conditions.
      (2) A single base change in the DNA results in a substitution of valine for glutamic acid in the sixth position of the globulin chain.
      (3) The Hb S gene is present in 10% of African-Americans
      (4) Etiologies
        (a) Sickle cell anemia
          ‣ Homozygous for HbSS
          ‣ Hemoglobin electrophoretic pattern
            • Hb S...........85-95%
            • Hb F.............5-15%
        (b) Sickling syndromes
          ‣ Double heterozygous

        • HbS-beta thalassemia

        • Hemoglobin SC disease

  (c) Sickle cell trait

     ▸ Heterozygous for HbS

     ▸ Hemoglobin electrophoretic pattern

       • Hb S...........40-45%

       • Hb A.........55-60%

     ▸ Clinically asymptomatic

     ▸ At risk for sudden death following vigorous exercise

b. DIAGNOSIS

  (1) History and physical findings in sickle cell anemia

    (a) Acute pain syndromes

     ▸ Vasoocclusive pain crisis

       • The most common manifestation of disease

       • Moderate → severe pain in the back extremities, ribs, and abdomen

       • ± precipitating factors

         ○ Dehydration

         ○ Infection

         ○ Physical or emotional stress

       • ± fever, leukocytosis, joint effusion

     ▸ Acute chest syndrome

       • Mild → severe → life-threatening

       • Precipitating factors

         ○ Embolism ± infarctions

          · Pulmonary

          · Sternum or ribs

         ○ Pneumonia

       • ↓ hemoglobin with chest pain, dyspnea, fever, pulmonary infiltrate and hypoxemia

     ▸ Splenic sequestration

       • Mild → severe → life-threatening

       • ↑ size of the spleen and ↓ in the hemoglobin

       • Infants and children most vulnerable

       • It is a sickle cell microvasculopathy

     ▸ Hand-foot syndrome

       • Infants and children most vulnerable

       • Swelling of one or more of the limbs

       • ± fever, leukocytosis

- Acute hepatic sequestration
    - ↑ size of the liver and ↓ in the hemoglobin
    - Acute hepatic crisis
        - Mild → severe → life-threatening
        - ↑ RUQ pain with ↑ hepatomegaly
        - ↑ of indirect bilirubin with ↑ of GGTP
        - ↑ PT and PTT
- Priapism

(b) Chronic pain syndromes
- Osteonecrosis
    Involvement of the femoral or humeral head
- Leg ulcers

(c) Infections
- Predilection to encapsulated organisms
    - *Streptococcus pneumoniae*
    - *Hemophilus influenzae*
- Osteomyelitis
    - *Salmonella* sp.
    - *Staphylococcus aureus*

(d) Organ failure
- CNS
    - CVA
- Heart
    - CHF
    - Cardiomegaly
    - High-output failure
- Kidney
    - Renal tubular defects
- Eyes
    - Proliferative retinopathy
    - Vitreous hemorrhage
    - Retinal detachment

(2) Laboratory
(a) Sickle cell anemia
- CBC
    - Hemoglobin ≈6-8 gm/dL
    - ↑ to normal WBCs and platelets
- Peripheral smear
    - Sickle cells

- Chem-28
    - ↑ LDH
    - ↑ bilirubin
- ↓ haptoglobin
- + sickledex

c. TREATMENT

(1) **Prevent dehydration and hypoxia**

(2) Acute chest syndrome

    (a) Correct the precipitating factors, if possible

    (b) IV and oral fluids

    (c) Correction of acidosis

    (d) Analgesics

    (e) Oxygen

(3) Acute chest syndrome

    (a) Hospitalization

    (b) Oxygen

    (c) Empiric antibiotic therapy

    (d) ± transfusion

    (e) Heparin for pulmonary embolism

(4) Splenic sequestration

    (a) Hemodynamic support

    (b) Transfusion

(5) Acute hepatic crisis

    Exchange transfusion

(6) Priapism

    (a) Hydration

    (b) Analgesics

    (c) ± transfusion

(7) Osteonecrosis

    (a) Analgesics

    (b) ↓ weight bearing

(8) Immunizations

    (a) Childhood immunizations

    (b) Pneumococcal vaccine

    (c) Hepatitis B vaccine

d. COMPLICATIONS

(1) Changes secondary to hemolysis

    (a) Cholelithiasis

    (b) Aplastic crisis

    (c) Folic acid deficiency

II. **WHITE BLOOD CELL DISORDERS**

A. *Chronic Lymphocytic Leukemia*

    1. DEFINITION

        a. The malignant proliferation of abnormal B-cell lymphocytes >95% of the time

        b. The most common leukemia in western countries.

        c. Patients age >50 years ≈90% of the time

    2. DIAGNOSIS

        a. History and Physical

            (1) Chronic fatigue

            (2) ↓ exercise tolerance

            (3) Pallor

            (4) Weight loss

            (5) Bruising

            (6) Lymphadenopathy

            (7) Splenomegaly

            (8) Hepatomegaly

        b. Laboratory

            (1) CBC

                (a) Red blood cells

                    Anemia

                (b) White blood cells

                    ▸ Mature appearing lymphocytes >10,000-200,000/μL

                    ▸ ± thrombocytopenia

                    ▸ Normal granulocytes

            (2) Bone marrow biopsy

                ≥30% lymphocytes

    3. TREATMENT

        a. No treatment of asymptomatic stable patients

        b. Chemotherapy

            (1) Chlorambucil

            (2) Cyclophosphamide

            (3) Prednisone

        c. Radiation therapy

            To ↓ bulky nodal or extranodal disease

        d. Surgery

            Splenectomy

    4. PROGNOSIS

        a. Survival with CLL is correlated to the stage at the time of diagnosis.

            (1) Stage 0............≈10.0 years

            (2) Stage I.............≈7.0 years

(3) Stage II.............$\approx$ 7.0 years

(4) Stage III............$\approx$ 2.0 years

(5) Stage IV............$\approx$ 2.0 years

B. *Chronic Myelogenous (Granulocytic) Leukemia*

1. DEFINITION

a. A malignant proliferation of abnormal granulocytic cells.

b. CML $\approx$20% of adult leukemias

c. Ph^1 chromosome is present $\approx$90% of the time

d. The prognosis is worse for Ph^1 negative leukemia.

2. DIAGNOSIS

a. **Chronic phase**

(1) Fatigue and malaise

(2) Weight loss

(3) $\pm$ fever and night sweats

(4) Leukocytosis

(5) Hepatosplenomegaly

(6) Bone pain

(7) Bruising

b. **Accelerated phase**

(1) A therapy resistant stage occurring $\approx$15% of the time

(2) Fever

(3) Weight loss

(4) Anorexia

(5) ↑ splenomegaly

(6) Anemia

(7) Thrombocytopenia

c. **Acute phase (Blast crisis)**

(1) Blast crisis

$\geq$30% of the myeloid cells in the marrow or blood are myeloblasts or promyelocytes.

(2) It may follow the accelerated phase *or* directly from the chronic phase.

(3) Signs and symptoms

(a) Fever

(b) Weight loss

(c) ↑ lymphadenopathy

(d) ↑ splenomegaly

(e) ↑ bone pain

(f) ↑ incidence of hemorrhage

(g) ↑ incidence of infection

(h) Meningeal leukemia

(4) Laboratory

  (a) CBC

     ▸ Anemia

       Normocytic, normochromic

     ▸ Leukocytosis

       • 30,000-300,000/μ/L

       • Thrombocytosis $\approx$50% of the time

     ▸ Peripheral smear

       Resembles the cellularity of a bone marrow biopsy

  (b) Bone marrow biopsy

     Hypercellular with an ↑ of the myeloid-erythroid ratio

  (c) NAP (Neutrophil alkaline phosphatase)

     Markedly ↓ or absent

  (d) Ph^1 chromosome

     Usually +

3. TREATMENT

  a. Chemotherapy

    (1) Bisulfan

    (2) Hydroxyurea

    (3) Interferon therapy

    (4) Bone marrow transplantation

  b. Allopurinol

    ↑ cellular turnover → ↑ uric acid

4. PROGNOSIS

  a. Mean survival following diagnosis of Ph^1-positive CML

    30-45 months

C. *Acute Lymphocytic Leukemia*

  1. DEFINITION

    a. A malignant proliferation of an early hematopoietic precursor yielding immature lymphoid cells referred to as blasts

    b. Affects children $\approx$80% of the time

    c. 3 subtypes L1, L2, L3 by morphology

  2. DIAGNOSIS

    a. History and Physical

      (1) Fatigue

      (2) Weight loss

      (3) Fever

      (4) Pallor

      (5) Petechiae and purpura

      (6) Bony pain

(7) Lymphadenopathy

(8) Hepatosplenomegaly

(9) CNS

    (a) Nausea and vomiting

    (b) Headache

    (c) Meningismus

(10) Gingival enlargement

b. Laboratory

    (1) Bone marrow biopsy

        (a) Hypercellularity + monotonous infiltration of immature

        (b) $\geq$30% blasts

    (2) CBC

        (a) Normocytic, normochromic anemia

        (b) Thrombocytopenia

        (c) WBC count

            ▸ ↑ in >50% of the cases.

    (3) Peripheral smear

        Blasts are identified

    (4) Cytochemical and immunologic markers differentiate subtypes.

3. TREATMENT

a. Remission-induction

    (1) Vincristine

    (2) Prednisone

    (3) ± L-asparaginase

    (4) ± daunorubicin

b. Maintenance

    (1) Methotrexate

    (2) Mercaptopurine

4. PROGNOSIS

a. Children

    $\approx$50-60% probable cure rate

b. Adults and adolescents

    $\approx$18-24 months

5. COMPLICATIONS

a. Hemorrhage

b. Infection

D. *Acute Myelogenous Leukemia*

1. DEFINITION

a. A malignant proliferation of an early hematopoietic precursor yielding immature myeloid cells referred to as blasts.

       b. Affects adults ≈90% of the time

       c. 7 subtypes M1-M7 by morphology

2. DIAGNOSIS

       a. History and Physical

           (1) Fatigue

           (2) Weight loss

           (3) Fever

           (4) Petechiae and purpura

           (5) ± bony pain

           (6) ± lymphadenopathy

           (7) ± hepatosplenomegaly

           (8) CNS

                 (a) + in subtypes M4,M5

                      ▸ Nausea and vomiting

                      ▸ Headache

                      ▸ Meningismus

       b. Laboratory

           (1) Bone marrow biopsy

                 (a) Hypercellularity + monotonous infiltration of immature cells

                 (b) ≥30% blasts

           (2) CBC

                 (a) Normocytic, normochromic anemia

                 (b) Thrombocytopenia

                 (c) WBC count ↑ in >50% of the cases.

           (3) Peripheral smear

               Blasts are identified

           (4) Cytochemical and quantitative bone marrow differential, help differentiate subtypes.

           (5) **Auer rods**

               Abnormal cytoplasmic granules

3. TREATMENT

       a. Remission-induction

           (1) Cytarabine

           (2) Idarubicin

       b. Postremission chemotherapy

           Cytarabine

       c. Bone marrow transplant

4. PROGNOSIS

       a. Mean survival in patients who achieve complete remission is ≈12-24 months

       b. 5-year survival ≈5-15% and probable cure

5. COMPLICATIONS
    a. Hemorrhage
    b. Infection
E. *Multiple (Plasma cell) Myeloma*
    1. DEFINITION
        The malignant proliferation of a single clone of plasma cells producing a monoclonal immunoglobulin.
    2. DIAGNOSIS
        a. History and Physical
            (1) Skeletal pain
            (2) Fatigue
            (3) Weakness
            (4) Weight loss
            (5) Hemorrhage
            (6) Recurrent infections
            (7) Renal insufficiency or failure
            (8) **Classic Triad**
                (a) Lytic bone lesions
                (b) Serum and/or urine monoclonal (M) protein
                (c) Marrow plasma cells >10%
            (9) Plasmacytoma
                (a) Usually skeletal in location
                (b) Monoclonal spike in serum and urine ≈50% of the time
        b. Laboratory
            (1) CBC
                Normochromic, normocytic anemia
            (2) Serum protein electrophoresis
                (a) IgG Monoclonal protein.............. ≈52% of the time
                (b) IgA Monoclonal protein.............. ≈22% of the time
                (c) Light chain only (Bence-Jones).... ≈25% of the time
            (3) Urine immunoelectrophoresis
                + for monoclonal protein≈80% of the time
            (4) 99% of patients have a monoclonal (M) protein in their urine or serum at the time of diagnosis.
            (5) X-ray examination
                (a) Punched out lesions
                (b) Pathologic fractures
            (6) Bone marrow biopsy
                >20% plasma cells

(7) Chem-28

Hypercalcemia

3. TREATMENT

a. Chemotherapy

(1) Melphalan

(2) Prednisone

b. Radiation therapy

Palliative

4. PROGNOSIS

a. Median survival for all patients is≈2-3 years months

b. Some patients survive >10 years

5. COMPLICATIONS

a. Hypercalcemia

b. Renal disease

(1) myeloma kidney

(2) Amyloidosis

c. Neurologic disease

(1) Spinal cord compression secondary to vertebral collapse

(2) Peripheral neuropathy

d. Infection

e. Hyperviscosity syndrome

III. LYMPHOMA

A. *Hodgkin's Disease*

1. DEFINITION

A malignant disease of lymphoid tissue which usually arises in the lymph nodes.

2. DIAGNOSIS

a. History and Physical

(1) **Painless lymphadenopathy**

(2) Fever

± Pel-Ebstein fever

(3) Night sweats

(4) Weight loss

(5) Fatigue and malaise

(6) Pruritus

(7) Hepatosplenomegaly

(8) Abdominal mass

(9) Pain

(a) Alcohol-induced pain

(b) Bone pain

b. Laboratory
    (1) **Lymph node biopsy**
        (a) Avoid the inguinal nodes if possible
        (b) Touch prep
        (c) Immunologic phenotyping
        (d) Electron microscopy
        (e) Cytogenetics
        (f) Molecular genetic analysis
    (2) Histology
        (a) **Reed-Sternberg cell**
            Pathognomonic of Hodgkin's
        (b) Rye Classification
           ‣ Lymphocyte predominant...................≈5%
           ‣ Nodular sclerosis........................≈65-80%
           ‣ Mixed cellularity.........................≈20-35%
           ‣ Lymphocyte depletion........................<5%
    (3) Chest X-ray
        Evaluation for mediastinal and/or hilar adenopathy
    (4) CT scan of chest and/or abdomen
        Evaluation of retroperitoneal, mesenteric and portal adenopathy
c. Cotswolds staging classification
    (1) Stage I
        Involvement of a single lymph node region or lymphoid structure
    (2) Stage II
        Involvement of two or more lymph node regions *on the same side of the diaphragm.*
    (3) Stage III
        Involvement of lymph node regions on both sides of the diaphragm
    (4) Stage IV
        Involvement of one or more extranodal sites in addition to a site for which the designation "E" has been used
d. Modifying factors
    (1) A = No systemic symptoms
    (2) B = Systemic symptoms
        (a) Fever
        (b) Night sweats
        (c) Weight loss
    (3) X = Bulky disease
    (4) E = Involvement of a single extranodal site that is contiguous or proximal to a known nodal site

3. TREATMENT
    a. Surgery
        (1) Biopsy
        (2) Staging laparotomy
    b. Radiation Therapy
    c. Chemotherapy
        (1) "MOPP"
            (a) Mechlorethamine
            (b) Oncovin (Vincristine)
            (c) Procarbazine
            (d) Prednisone
        (2) "ABVD"
            (a) Adriamycin
            (b) Bleomycin
            (c) Vinblastine
            (d) Dacarbazine
4. PROGNOSIS
    Current therapy cures >70% of patients.

I. **PELVIC INFLAMMATORY DISEASE**
  A. DEFINITION
    1. An *ascending infection* from the vagina or endocervix affecting the uterus, fallopian tubes, ovaries and broad ligaments
    2. Salpingitis and salpingo-oophoritis are synonymous terms
    3. Ascending infection causes ≈99% of pelvic inflammatory disease
    4. Primary
      a. Usually sexually transmitted
      b. Etiologies
        (1) *Neisseria gonorrhoeae*
        (2) *Chlamydia trachomatis*
        (3) Anaerobes
          (a) *Bacteroides* spp.
          (b) *Peptostreptococcus* spp.
          (c) *Peptococcus* spp.
        (4) Facultative
          (a) *E coli*
          (b) *Streptococcus* spp.
          (c) *Hemophilus influenzae*
          (d) *Gardnerella vaginalis*
        (5) Mycoplasma (controversial)
          (a) *Mycoplasma hominis*
          (b) *Ureaplasma urealyticum*
    5. Secondary
      Intrauterine procedure or surgery
  B. DIAGNOSIS
    1. History and Physical
      a. Pelvic pain
      b. Leukorrhea
      c. Fever
      d. Abnormal vaginal bleeding
      e. ↑ pain to palpation to pelvic organs
      f. ↑ pain to movement of cervix
      g. Discharge from the cervix
    2. Laboratory
      a. CBC
        Leukocytosis
      b. ↑ sedimentation rate
      c. Gram stain of cervical secretions
        Nearly 50% of the time *gram-negative* intracellular diplococci (gonorrhea)
      d. Cervical culture
        Identification of organism(s)

e. β-hCG

(1) Rule out ectopic pregnancy

(2) Determine pregnancy status before treatment

f. ± pelvic ultrasound

Assess fallopian tubes and ovaries for signs of infection.

g. Laparoscopy

Reserved in cases when diagnosis is clouded or a failure of therapy

C. TREATMENT

1. Most protocols are dependent upon the organism(s) isolated.

2. Empiric

a. Outpatient

Ceftriaxone 250 mg IM *followed by* **doxycycline 100 mg PO x 14 days**

b. Inpatient

Cefoxitin 2.0 g. IV QID or cefotetan 2.0 g IV BID + doxycycline 100 mg bid for at least 48 hrs *after* the patient improves, then continue the doxy-cycline for a total of 14 days or therapy.

3. Evaluate and treat sexual partner(s)

4. Test of cure following completion of therapy

5. Ambulatory patients who don't respond to treatment within 72 hours should be hospitalized

II. SYPHILIS

A. DEFINITION

An infection caused by the spirochete *Treponema pallidum*.

B. DIAGNOSIS

1. Syphilis is classified by stages

a. **Primary**

(1) **Chancre**

(a) ≈10-90 days after exposure.

(b) A painless papule ulcerates forming an indurated lesion with a smooth base and firm borders.

(2) ± regional lymphadenopathy

(3) Chancre *heals* within 3-6 weeks

b. **Secondary**

(1) Begins 6-8 weeks following the presentation of the chancre

(2) Nonspecific complaints

(a) Malaise

(b) Fatigue

(c) Headache

(d) Fever

(e) Sore throat

(3) Generalized lymphadenopathy

(4) Generalized maculopapular rash which progresses to a papular rash most pronounced on the palms and soles.

(5) **Condyloma lata**

    (a) Papules which coalesce forming large, flat, *highly infectious* lesions on moist areas and genitals

    (b) Highly infectious lesions can occur on mucous membranes

(6) Systemic manifestations *may* occur

    (a) Hepatitis

    (b) Periostitis

    (c) Nephropathy

    (d) Uveitis/iritis

clinical signs of syphilis

ebrospinal fluid is normal

ly latency

The first year after infection

e latency

(a) Latent infection >1 year

(b) Not infectious *except*

      ‣ Pregnancy

      ‣ Transfusion

benign syphilis (Gumma)

a) May form 1-10 years after initial infection.

b) Destructive granulomatous lesions that can affect any area of the body

c) They respond rapidly to treatment

iovascular syphilis

) Begins 5-10 years after initial infection.

) Clinically seen 20-30 years after primary infection.

) An obliterative endarteritis of the vasa vasorum

) Usually involves the *ascending aorta* manifest as aortic insuffic-iency and/or aortic aneurysm.

syphilis

(a) Asymptomatic

    + VDRL in CSF

(b) Meningovascular

      ‣ Begins 5-10 years after initial infection

      ‣ Acute or subacute aseptic meningitis

           (c) Tabes dorsalis
- 20-30 years after initial infection
- Progressive degeneration of the posterior roots and columns of the spinal cord.
- Charcot's joints
- Argyll-Robertson pupils

           (d) General paresis
- Chronic meningo-encephalitis which evolves into a syphilitic psychosis

2. Laboratory
- a. Darkfield examination
  - (1) + In *primary* syphilis
  - (2) + In moist mucosal lesions of secondary syphilis
- b. VDRL (Venereal disease research lab test)
  - (1) Nonspecific anticardiolipin antibodies by slide flocculation
    - (a) Screening
    - (b) Quantitation
- c. RPR (Rapid plasma reagin test)
  - (1) Nonspecific anticardiolipin antibodies by agglutination
  - (2) Screening
- d. FTA-ABS
  - (1) Immunofluorescence with absorbed serum
  - (2) Confirmatory test

C. TREATMENT
1. General
- a. Jarisch-Herxheimer reaction
  - (1) Fever, ± adenopathy, ± skin rash, arthralgias six hours post therapy.
  - (2) It lasts about 24 hours.
- b. **Treponemal resistance to erythromycin has been documented.**

2. Incubating

        Ceftriaxone 250 mg IM *followed by* **Doxycycline 100 mg x 10 days**

3. Primary, Secondary, Early latent
- a. 2.4 million units of *Benzathine penicillin* IM or for PCN allergy
- b. Vibramycin 100 mg BID x 15 days or
- c. Ceftriaxone 250 mg IM x 10 days

4. Late latent, Late benign, Cardiovascular
- a. 2.4 million units of *Benzathine penicillin* IM weekly for *three successive weeks* for a total of 7.2 million units or for PCN allergy
- b. Vibramycin 100 mg BID x 30 days.

5. Neurosyphilis

    a. 2-4 million units of aqueous penicillin IV every 4 hours x 10 days or

    b. 2-4 million units of procaine penicillin *IM* + probenicid 500 mg QID daily x 15 days.

III. **ROCKY MOUNTAIN SPOTTED FEVER**

  A. DEFINITION

    1. An acute febrile illness most often characterized by a rickettsia-induced vasculitis.

    2. Etiology

      Rickettsia rickettsii

    3. In the United States the vector and principal reservoir are ixodid ticks

      a. *Dermacentor andersoni,* the Rocky Mountain wood tick

      b. *Dermocentor variabilis,* the American dog tick

  B. DIAGNOSIS

    1. History and physical

      a. Early symptoms are nonspecific

        (1) Fever

        (2) Headache

        (3) Malaise

        (4) Myalgias

      b. **A classic maculopapular or petechial rash**

        (1) Three to seven days following exposure

        (2) *Initially* involving the hands and feet (palms and soles)

        (3) ± centripetal movement of rash

      c. Gastrointestinal

        (1) Abdominal pain

        (2) Nausea, vomiting and diarrhea

      d. Neurological

        (1) Seizures

        (2) Confusion

      e. Late symptoms

        (1) Pneumonia

        (2) DIC

    2. Laboratory

      a. CBC

        (1) WBC and differential are normal

        (2) Thrombocytopenia

      b. Complement fixation and Weil-Felix tests not + until the 8-12 day

      c. Fluorescent antibody stains of the skin or tissues + as early as day 4

  C. TREATMENT

    1. Doxycycline

2. Chloramphenicol

3. **Always initiate therapy *early* if there is a high index of clinical suspicion.**

IV. **LYME DISEASE**
    A. DEFINITION
        1. A spirochetal infection causing multisystemic illness spread by the tick of the *Ixodes* genus.
        2. Etiology
            The spirochete *Borrelia burgdorferi*
    B. DIAGNOSIS
        1. Stage 1 is characterized by local infection
            a **Erythema migrans** at the site of the tick bite.
                (1) Incubation ≈ three days to one month
                (2) Initially a red macule or papule that enlarges to form a larger annular lesion often characterized by an erythematous border and partial central clearing.
                (3) Common sites
                    (a) Axilla
                    (b) Thigh
                    (c) Groin
        2. Stage 2 is characterized by disseminated infection
            a. Occurring days *after* the onset of erythema migrans
            b. Constitutional symptoms
                (1) **Fatigue and malaise**
                (2) Fever and chills
                (3) Severe headache
            c. Arthralgias
            d. **Migratory musculoskeletal pain**
            e. Annular skin lesions
            f. Less common manifestations
                (1) Generalized lymphadenopathy
                (2) Splenomegaly
                (3) Hepatitis
            g. Fatigue and malaise are continuous with other signs and symptoms intermittent.
            h. Early signs and symptoms disappear or markedly improve after several weeks even without treatment.
            i. Neurologic symptoms develop in ≈15% of patients
                (1) Weeks to months following the initial infection,.the most common pattern of involvement includes variable signs and symptoms of meningitis associated with a facial palsy and a peripheral radiculoneuropathy.
                (2) Neurologic signs and symptoms totally resolve within months but chronic forms may present later.

j. Cardiovascular disease develops in ≈8% of patients.

Most commonly AV block

3. Stage 3 is characterized by persistent infection

a. **Arthritis**

Large joints, commonly knees.

b. Less common

Chronic skin or neurologic disease.

4. Laboratory

a. Clinical diagnosis + serological confirmation

(1) ELISA

(2) Immunoblot test

C. TREATMENT

1. Stage 1

a. Ten days of antibiotic therapy is adequate.

(1) Doxycycline

Do not give pregnant women or children tetracyclines or their derivatives.

(2) Amoxicillin

(3) Cefuroxime

(4) Erythromycin is *less* effective

2. Disseminated disease

a. Twenty to thirty days of therapy is indicated

b. Lyme arthritis

(1) 30 days of antibiotic therapy may be effective

(2) A small group will not respond to antibiotic therapy and a synovectomy may be indicated.

c. Neurologic and cardiovascular disease

(1) Parenteral antibiotics

(a) Cefuroxime

(b) Penicillin

(2) ± corticosteroids

V. **RUBEOLA**

A. DEFINITION

1. Measles is a highly infectious viral illness characterized by an acute febrile eruption.

2. Infected individuals are contagious five days after exposure to five days after the rash has appeared.

3. From exposure to first symptoms ≈8-12 days with the rash appearing at 14 days.

B. DIAGNOSIS
  1. Prodromal stage (3-4 days)
      a. Fever
      b. Malaise
      c. Irritability
      d. Conjunctivitis
      e. Photophobia
      f. Severe cough
      g. Runny nose
      h. **Koplik's spots**
          They appear on mucous membranes of the mouth 1-2 days before the onset of the rash and are characterized as small, irregular, red lesions with a blue-white center.
  2. Eruptive Stage
      a. An erythematous, maculopapular rash appears on the forehead which spreads downward toward the feet over a period of 3 days.
      b. The total duration of the rash is ≈6 days.
      c. Most of the prodromal symptoms *except cough* disappear 24-48 hours following the onset of the rash.
  3. Laboratory
      a. Leukopenia is common during the prodrome.
      b. A leukocytosis indicates a complication such as superinfection.
      c. Multinucleated giant cells can be identified in stained preps of sputum and urine.
      d. Multiple serologic tests are available for confirmation.
C. TREATMENT
  1. No therapy is indicated for uncomplicated measles.
  2. Active immunity is induced with a live, attenuated measles vaccine if patients are innoculated *after* 15 months of age.
D. COMPLICATIONS
  1. Superimposed bacterial infections
      a. Pneumonia
      b. Bilateral otitis media
  2. Conjunctivitis which progresses to corneal ulceration or keratitis
  3. Myocarditis
  4. Encephalomyelitis
  5. Thrombocytopenia
  6. Rare complications
      a. Interstitial giant cell pneumonia
          Associated with malnutrition or immunodeficiency
      b. Subacute sclerosing panencephalitis

VI. **MUMPS**

A. DEFINITION

1. An communicable viral illness most often characterized by painful swelling in the parotid and other salivary glands.

2. Illness in a nonimmunized individual occurs within 2-3 weeks of exposure.

3. Mumps virus may also cause

a. Epididymo-orchitis

(1) Uncommon in children but up to ≈25% in postpubertal males.

(2) Occurs a week to ten days following the parotitis.

b. Pancreatitis

c. Aseptic meningitis

d. Encephalitis

e. Less commonly

(1) Oophoritis

(2) Thyroiditis

(3) Migratory polyarthritis

B. DIAGNOSIS

1. The diagnosis is usually made on clinical grounds alone.

2. Prodrome

a. Fever

b. Malaise

c. Anorexia

3. **Painful parotid gland swelling**

a. Bilateral parotid gland swelling in ≈66% of cases

b. Other salivary glands involved ≈10% of cases

4. Laboratory

a. Mumps-IgM antibody

b. Isolation of the virus from the throat or from saliva

C. TREATMENT

Mumps runs its course in 7-10 days.

VII. **RUBELLA**

A. DEFINITION

1. A benign, febrile viral exanthem also known as "Three day measles" or "German measles".

2. It is not as contagious as measles.

a. **Congenital rubella**

(1) If infection occurs in a pregnant woman profound fetal malformation and chronic fetal infection may occur.

(a) Deafness

(b) Microcephaly

(c) Mental retardation

(d) Cardiovascular malformations

(e) Ophthalmologic malformations

B. DIAGNOSIS

1. Prodrome presents 1-7 days *before* the exanthem.

    a. Fever

    b. Headache

    c. Malaise

    d. Conjunctivitis

    e. Lymphadenopathy

2. A maculopapular rash appears on the face and spreads downward to the abdomen and legs.

3. The rash presents 2-3 weeks following exposure and usually resolves in three or so days.

4. Arthralgias may occur

5. Certain diagnosis of rubella is by virus isolation and identification *or* by changes in antibody titer.

C. TREATMENT

1. Supportive therapy is the usual.

2. Gamma globulin may prevent clinical disease however transplacental transmission of the virus may still occur.

3. Live, attenuated rubella vaccine provides active immunization

4. **Never give rubella vaccine to a pregnant woman *or* a woman who wishes to conceive within 90 days of conception.**

VIII. **Varicella-Zoster**

A. DEFINITION

1. There are two distinct clinical entities.

    a. **Varicella = Chickenpox**

        A *childhood illness* which is highly contagious and characterized by an erythmatous, vesicular rash.

    b. **Herpes Zoster = Shingles**

        (1) An *adult* illness usually occurring in the later years of life in the immunocompetent individual.

        (2) Infection represents a *reactivation* of the latent varicella-zoster virus which is characterized as a painful, vesicular rash.

        (3) Zoster involves *dermatomes*.

        (4) Reactivation of a latent Varicella-Zoster virus in the dorsal root ganglia occurs with migration of the virus along the *sensory nerves* to the skin.

B. DIAGNOSIS

    1. Chickenpox

        a. Incubation following exposure is 1-17 days

        b. Low-grade fever

        c. Malaise

        d. **Rash**

            (1) Papules → vesicles → pustules → crusting → resolution

            (2) Initially on the face and trunk and then can involve the entire body.

    2. Zoster

        a. Prodrome

            (1) ≈5 days of dysesthesia or radicular pain *before* the vesicular eruption

            (2) The vesicular rash is usually unilateral and doesn't cross the midline

            (3) Multiple contiguous dermatomes may be involved

        b. Triggering factors

            (1) Immunosuppression

            (2) Increasing age

            (3) Trauma including surgery

            (4) ± stress

        c. Laboratory

            (1) Tzanck smear of skin lesions

            (2) Cultures of skin lesions

            (3) Gram stain to differentiate from folliculitis or impetigo.

C. TREATMENT

    1. **Avoid aspirin and aspirin-like medications because of the ↑ development of Reye's syndrome.**

    2. Chickenpox

        a. Immunocompetent patients

            (1) Antipruritics

            (2) Adequate skin care to prevent secondary infection

            (3) Oral acyclovir therapy for severe cases

        b. Immunocompromised patients

            IV acyclovir

    3. Shingles

        a. Immunocompetent patients

            (1) Analgesics to control the acute neuritis or postherpetic neuritis.

            (2) Adequate skin care to prevent secondary infection

            (3) Oral acyclovir therapy

            (4) Oral valacyclovir

        b. Immunocompromised patients

            IV acyclovir

D. COMPLICATIONS
1. Shingles
Postherpetic neuralgia
2. **Varicella-Zoster infection in an immunocompromised patient can be deadly.**

IX. INFECTIOUS MONONUCLEOSIS
A. DEFINITION
An infectious disease caused by the Epstein-Barr virus
B. DIAGNOSIS
1. History and physical
a. Sore throat
b. Fever
c. Lymphadenopathy
d. ± headache
e. ± rash
f. ± splenomegaly
2. Laboratory
a. CBC
Atypical lymphocytosis
b. + heterophile antibody testing
C. TREATMENT
a. Rest
b. Supportive care
c. Check for co-infection and guard against secondary infection
d. ± glucocorticoids
e. Rash occurs when ampicillin is used in a patient with Ebstein-Barr infection

X. ACQUIRED IMMUNE DEFICIENCY SYNDROME
A. DEFINITION
1. An infection caused by an RNA virus that produces profound immunologic defects.
2. **AIDS is spread by intimate sexual contact or by parenteral contact with blood or body fluids.**
B. DIAGNOSIS
1. HIV screening with ELISA
2. A positive screen should must be confirmed with a Western blot test.
3. **Indicator conditions in case definition of AIDS**
a. Fungal infections
(1) Candidiasis
(a) Esophagus
(b) Trachea

(c) Bronchi

(d) Lungs

(2) Cryptococcal infection, *extrapulmonary*

b. Protozoan infections

(1) ***Pneumocystis carinii***

(2) Cryptosporidiosis with associated diarrhea >1 month

(3) Toxoplasmosis, disseminated (excluding congenital infection)

c. Mycobacterial infections

(1) *Mycobacterium avium*, disseminated

(2) *Mycobacterium* kansasii, disseminated

d. Helminthic infection

Strongyloidiasis (extraintestinal)

e. Viral infection (excluding congenital infection)

(1) Cytomegalovirus of any organ excluding the liver, spleen or lymph nodes

(2) Herpes simplex

(a) Mucocutaneous ulcer >1 month

(b) Esophagitis

(c) Bronchitis

(d) Pneumonia

(3) Progressive multifocal leukoencephalopathy secondary to JC virus

f. Malignancy

(1) Kaposi's sarcoma in a patient <60 years of age

(2) Primary lymphoma of the brain <60 years of age

g. Neuropsychiatric disease

HIV encephalopathy

4. **Indicator conditions in case definition of AIDS** *requiring positive HIV serology.*

a. A CD4 T lymphocyte count <200 cells per cubic millimeter

b. Fungal infections

(1) Coccidioidomycosis, disseminated

(2) Histoplasmosis, disseminated

(3) Nocardiosis

c. Protozoan infections

Isosporosis with diarrhea

d. Mycobacterial infections

Mycobacterium tuberculosis

e. Bacterial infections

(1) Recurrent bacterial pneumonia

(2) Recurrent Salmonella septicemia (non-typhoid)

f. Malignancy

(1) Invasive cervical cancer

(2) Kaposi's sarcoma in a patient >60 years of age

(3) Primary lymphoma of the brain >60 years of age

(4) High-grade B cell non-Hodgkin's lymphoma

(5) Non-Hodgkin's lymphoma, undifferentiated

(6) Immunoblastic lymphoma

  g. Organ-specific disease

    Lymphoid interstitial pneumonia and/or pulmonary lymphoid hyperplasia in a child <13 years of age.

  h. Miscellaneous

    HIV wasting syndrome

  5. Risk for specific infection is related to the circulating CD4+ count

    a. CD4+ lymphocyte count <500/microliter

      Mycobacterium tuberculosis

    b. CD4+ lymphocyte count <200/microliter

      (1) *Pneumocystis carinii*

      (2) *Histoplasma capsulatum*

      (3) *Cryptococcus neoformans*

    c. CD4+ lymphocyte count <50/microliter

      Mycobacterium avium-intracellulare

C. TREATMENT

  1. Antiretroviral therapy

    a. Slows viral replication but does not kill the virus.

      (1) CD4 T lymphocytes count >500 cells/mm³

        No therapy.

      (2) CD4 T lymphocyte count between 200 and 500 cells/mm³

        (a) Some controversy exists

          ▸ Several U.S. studies show benefit to early therapy

          ▸ European studies failed to document benefit to early therapy

        (b) Begin therapy if

          ▸ The patient becomes symptomatic

          ▸ Has a history of opportunistic infections

      (3) CD4 T lymphocytes count <200 cells/mm³

        (a) Begin therapy

      (4) Always begin antiretroviral therapy if there is deterioration of the patient's condition as determined by laboratory or clinical findings.

  2. Treatment, suppression or prevention of opportunistic infections

    a. *Pneumocystis carinii*

      (1) DEFINITION

        (a) An infection of the lung parenchyma by the fungus *Pneumocystis carinii*.

        (b) It is the most common *opportunistic* infection in a patient with AIDS.

(2) DIAGNOSIS

    (a) Signs and symptoms
- Fever
- Cough
- Dyspnea
- Tachypnea

    (b) Pneumocystis may disseminate

    (c) Laboratory
- ***Pneumocystis carinii* has not been cultured**
- No reliable serologic tests
- Chest X-ray
  - Normal → diffuse *interstitial* infiltrates
- Diagnosis by examination of pulmonary secretions or lung biopsy
  - Sputum induction
  - Bronchoscopy
  - Bronchoalveolar lavage
  - Transbronchial biopsy

(3) TREATMENT

    (a) Trimethoprim-sulfamethoxazole

    (b) Pentamidine

    (c) Atovaquone

    (d) Dapsone-trimethoprim

b. Candidiasis

    (1) TREATMENT

        (a) Oral
- Nystatin solution or tablets
- Clotrimazole troches

        (b) Esophageal
- Fluconazole

c. Systemic mycoses

    (1) TREATMENT

        (a) Amphotericin B

        (b) Fluconazole

d. Cytomegalovirus

    (1) TREATMENT

        Ganciclovir

    e. *Herpes simplex*
       (1) TREATMENT
          Acyclovir
    f. Toxoplasmosis
       (1) TREATMENT
          Pyrimethamine + Sulfadiazine
    g. Tuberculosis
       (1) TREATMENT
          Isoniazid + Rifampin + Ethambutol + Pyrazinamide

XI. INFECTIOUS DIARRHEA
  A. DEFINITION
    1. Diarrhea
      Three or more poorly formed stools in 24 hrs hours
    2. Etiologies of infectious diarrhea
      a. Viral
        (1) Rotavirus
        (2) Norwalk virus
      b. Bacterial
        (1) *E coli*
        (2) *Salmonella* sp.
        (3) *Shigella* sp.
        (4) *Campylobacter* sp.
        (5) *Vibrio* sp.
        (6) *Yersinia enterocolitica*
      c. Parasitic
        (1) *Giardia lamblia*
        (2) *E histolytica*
        (3) *Cryptosporidium*
  B. DIAGNOSIS
    1. History and Physical
      a. Loose watery stools
        (1) ± blood
        (2) ± mucous
      b. Fever ± chills
      c. Nausea and vomiting
      d. Abdominal pain
      e. Bloating
      f. Dehydration

2. Laboratory
  a. Stool examination
    (1) Blood, ova and parasite
    (2) Fecal leukocytes
    (3) Stool cultures and sensitivity
  b. CBC
    (1) Leukocytosis
    (2) Dehydration
  c. Serum electrolytes
    Dehydration

C. TREATMENT
  1. Nonpharmacologic
    a. No caffeine, alcohol or dairy products
    b. ↑ fluids and salt
    c. Rest
  2. Pharmacologic
    a. IV fluids in severe disease
    b. Pepto-Bismol
    c. Viral
      Supportive care only
    d. Bacterial
      (1) *E coli*
        (a) Ciprofloxacin
        (b) Sulfamethoxazole-Trimethoprim
      (2) *Salmonella* spp.
        (a) No treatment unless *S typhi* or if septic
        (b) Ciprofloxacin
        (c) Sulfamethoxazole-Trimethoprim
      (3) *Shigella* spp.
        (a) Ciprofloxacin
        (b) Sulfamethoxazole-Trimethoprim
      (4) *Campylobacter* sp.
        (a) Erythromycin
        (b) Ciprofloxacin
      (5) *Vibrio* sp.
        Tetracycline
      (6) *Yersinia enterocolitica*
        (a) No treatment unless severe illness
        (b) Sulfamethoxazole-Trimethoprim

(7) *Clostridium difficile*
    (a) Metronidazole
    (b) Oral Vancomycin
e. Parasitic
    (1) *Giardia lamblia*
        Metronidazole
    (2) *E histolytica*
        Metronidazole
    (3) *Cryptosporidium*
        Paromomycin

1. A 10 year old boy presents with a rash on the left knee. The rash is vesiculopustular and has spread since it was first noticed five days earlier. Weeping lesions form shallow ulcers with "honey-colored crusts". The most likely diagnosis:
   - A. Herpes simplex
   - B. Contact dermatitis
   - C. Impetigo
   - D. Lymphangitis

2. The most likely etiology of this rash
   - A. Viral
   - B. Allergic
   - C. Bacterial
   - D. None of the above

3. The most appropriate treatment
   - A. Acyclovir
   - B. Topical steroids
   - C. Oral antibiotic therapy
   - D. Reassurance that the rash will clear spontaneously

4. Condylomata acuminata
   - A. The rash of secondary syphilis
   - B. The rash caused by human papilloma virus
   - C. Can undergo malignant transformation
   - D. Is not contagious

5. A 60 year old weathered cowboy presents with a pearly, translucent, smooth papule with rolled edges and surface telangiectasia on his forehead. "Been there for years but the thing is kind a growin'", he drawls. The most likely diagnosis:
   - A. Basal cell carcinoma
   - B. Squamous cell carcinoma
   - C. Melanoma
   - D. None of the above

6. "Momma told me I was growin' like a weed", says Hugo L., a 16 year old who is seven feet tall. " And I'm still growin", he laughs. You would expect:
   - A. Lytic bone lesions
   - B. Parathyroid adenona
   - C. Adrenal adenoma
   - D. None of the above

7. "All Melvin does is get after me all the time, moles, that's all I ever hear about", says Sadie, a 45 year old woman. "The fool tells me the thing is changing color and is growing", she sighs. Examination reveals an asymmetrical pigmented lesion with an irregular border about 1 cm in greatest transverse diameter. You should:
   - A. Reassure her that the mole is benign and that her husband is in need of psycho-therapy
   - B. Reassure her and recheck the lesion in three months
   - C. Biopsy the lesion
   - D. Treat the lesion with topical steroids and antibiotics for five weeks

8. Melanoma
   - A. Is a deadly tumor
   - B. Readily responds to chemotherapy
   - C. Usually arise from intradermal nevi
   - D. Two of the above
   - E. All of the above

9. A chronic lid inflammation of the glands surrounding the eyelashes
   - A. Chalazion
   - B. Blepharitis
   - C. Hordeolum
   - D. Conjunctivitis

10. A 60 year old man presents with an intraocular pressure of 30 mm Hg in the right eye and 26 mm Hg in the left eye. He also complains of visual field loss. These findings are consistent with a diagnosis of:
    - A. Cataracts
    - B. Hypertensive retinopathy
    - C. Diabetic retinopathy
    - D. None of the above

11. Treatment of this gentleman would include
    A. Immediate surgery
    B. Vasodilators and ACE inhibitors
    C. Topical anticholinergics
    D. None of the above

12. Aeration of the middle ear is essential in the treatment of otitis media *regardless* of stage.
    A. True
    B. False

13. A 4 year old girl presents with a one week history of ear pain. Upon examination you observe 100.5° F. temperature recorded orally, anterior cervical adenopathy, and a red, bulging tympanic membrane. The tympanic membrane is immobile by pneumatic otoscopy. White blood cell count is 14,500 cells mm³ with a shift to the left. You would:
    A. Suggest tympanoplasty tubes stat
    B. Oral antibiotic therapy for ten days and recheck
    C. Treat the ear canal with topical antibiotic steroid drops
    D. Work up the patient for leukemia

14. A 40 year old woman presents with unilateral tinnitus associated with hearing loss. She also complains of occasional vertigo. MRI reveals an acoustic neuroma. Appropriate treatment:
    A. Surgery
    B. Chemotherapy
    C. Two of the above
    D. All of the above

15. Complications of acute otitis media include
    A. Labyrinthitis
    B. Meningitis
    C. Extradural abscess
    D. Two of the above
    E. All of the above

16. A 36 year old man presents with an acute onset of submandibular swelling after eating a pickle. "Damn tender it is but the swellin' is goin' down a bit now, come to think of it". The most probable diagnosis:

A. Sialoadenitis
B. Sialolithiasis
C. Squamous cell carcinoma of the floor of the mouth
D. Two of the above
E. All of the above

17. A 3 year old comes in with a rapid onset of fever to 103° F. recorded orally, severe pharyngitis and respiratory distress associated with difficulty swallowing and drooling. You should:
    A. Immediately inspect the throat using a tongue depressor.
    B. Initiate therapy with racemic epinephrine and systemic steroids
    C. Place the patient on oral antibiotics and follow-up in a week to ten days.
    D. None of the above.

18. A 55 year old smoker presents with a 6 month history of hoarseness. Laryngoscopy reveals a tumor on the vocal cord. The most probable histologic typing of the tumor:
    A. Adenocarcinoma
    B. Basal cell carcinoma
    C. Squamous cell carcinoma
    D. Mixed tumor

19. A 44 year old woman presents with a three day history of fever, chills, headache associated with left chest pain and shortness of breath. While examining her she coughs up blood-tinged sputum. Auscultation of the lungs reveal bi-basilar crackles. Appropriate tests would include:
    A. Gram stain of the sputum
    B. CBC
    C. Chest X-ray
    D. Two of the above
    E. All of the above

20. Gram stain of the sputum reveals gram-positive encapsulated, elongated, paired cocci. The most probable etiology of the pneumonia:
    A. *Hemophilus influenzae*
    B. *Moraxella catarrhalis*

C. *Pseudomonas aeruginosa*

D. *Streptococcus pneumoniae*

21. Atypical pneumonias:
    A. Respond well to penicillins
    B. Are usually benign and self-limiting
    C. Are easily diagnosed with a Gram stain
    D. Two of the above
    E. None of the above

22. A 60 year old obese man presents stating, "I cough so hard I'm turnin' blue". His history reveals chronic productive cough and intermittent dyspnea for years. He has smoked a pack of cigarettes a day for over 40 years. Physical findings include bilateral rhonchi and wheezes, pedal edema, and cyanosis of the lips during a paroxysm of cough. Expected findings on chest X-ray:
    A. Increased brochovascular markings ± cardiomegaly
    B. A small heart with hyperinflation of the lungs, flat diaphragms and bullous changes
    C. ± hyperinflation, ± patchy infiltrates secondary to atelectasis
    D. Basilar fibrosis, pleural thickening and effusion

23. The most probable diagnosis:
    A. Chronic bronchitis
    B. Emphysema
    C. Asthma
    D. Interstitial lung disease

24. Appropriate treatment would include:
    A. Stop smoking
    B. Beta-blockers
    C. Theophyllines
    D. Two of the above
    E. All of the above

25. A 56 year old lady presents with an 8 month history of weight loss, increasing cough, dyspnea and occasional chest pain. "I'm quite worried, doctor, because I coughed up a bit of blood this morning",

she mutters. Chest X-ray reveals a 5 cm hilar mass. Statistically, the lesion should be:
    A. Non-small cell carcinoma
    B. Small cell carcinoma
    C. Asbestosis
    D. Sarcoidosis

26. Appropriate therapy may include:
    A. Surgery
    B. Radiation therapy
    C. Chemotherapy
    D. All of the above
    E. None of the above

27. The prognosis:
    A. Excellent with full and total recovery
    B. Good with vigorous treatment with systemic steroids and appropriate use of antibiotics
    C. Guarded but she should be able to carry on for decades
    D. Statistically poor with the majority of patient dying within 5 years of diagnosis.

28. A 23 year old female presents to the ER with dyspnea, tachypnea, anxiety, tachycardia, and chest pain. She has been under increased stress at work. She is on no medication except birth control pills. Physical examination reveals few findings except a low grade temperature and an accentuated P_2. CBC is normal, arterial blood gases are normal as are the chest X-ray and ECG. Your working diagnosis:
    A. Conversion reaction
    B. Early bronchitis and pleurisy
    C. Rule out pulmonary embolus
    D. Emphysema

29. Based on the diagnosis above, you should:
    A. Reassure the patient and discharge her with an anxiolytic for her stress.
    B. Start her on empiric antibiotic therapy to cover for probable bronchitis and pleurisy.

C. Order a V/Q (Ventilation/perfusion) lung scan

D. None of the above

30. A 62 year old man is diagnosed with silent ischemia. He should be treated even though he has no signs and symptoms of coronary artery disease.
    A. True
    B. False

31. Complications of high blood pressure include:
    A. Cerebrovascular accident
    B. Chronic renal disease
    C. Congestive heart failure
    D. Two of the above
    E. All of the above

32. A 66 year old man presents to the ER with a history of crushing substernal chest pain which radiates into his left arm and jaw. I been takin' my "nitros", he gasps, "but they're not working". He threw up on the way to the car and feels like he could pass out. Physical examination reveals a blood pressure of 160/100 mm Hg supine, a thready pulse of 120 beats/minute and respirations of 24/minute. He is diaphoretic. Auscultation reveals scattered wheezes and crackles, and a S_4. You note jugular vein distention. The most probable diagnosis:
    A. Acute myocardial infarction
    B. Pulmonary embolus
    C. Pneumonia
    D. Labile hypertension

33. Chest X-ray is non-specific, the ECG reveals non-specific ST-T wave changes. Chem-28 and CBC are normal. Blood gases are essentially normal. You should:
    A. Discharge him with instructions to increase his sublingual nitroglycerin and follow-up with his doctor in the morning.
    B. Add a thiazide diuretic to take care of the hypertension and send him home with some Tylenol with codeine.
    C. Admit to the hospital for monitoring and further evaluation

D. Order a V/Q (Ventilation/perfusion) lung scan and if normal discharge.

34. A 60 year old female presents complaining of an irregular pulse. On ECG, no P waves are identified and QRS are not evenly spaced. The diagnosis:
    A. Atrial fibrillation
    B. Atrial flutter
    C. Multifocal atrial tachycardia
    D. Ventricular premature contractions

35. The etiology of this arrhythmia include:
    A. Organic heart disease
    B. Hyperthyroidism
    C. COPD
    D. Two of the above
    E. All of the above

36. A 44 year old man presents with a history of 104° F. temperature, chills, night sweats and arthralgias. Physical exam reveals a B.P. of 134/94, a pulse of 110 beats/minute and regular and a temperature of 103.5° F. recorded orally. On auscultation, the patient has a regurgitant mitral valve murmur. Other physical findings include painless red nodules on the palms and soles, splinter hemorrhages, and painful reddish-purple lesions on the fingers. The most probable diagnosis:
    A. Acute rheumatic fever
    B. Infective endocarditis
    C. Acute pericarditis
    D. Hypertrophic cardiomyopathy

37. Appropriate laboratory testing would include:
    A. CBC
    B. Blood cultures
    C. Echocardiography
    D. All of the above

38. All of the following are major manifestations of acute rheumatic fever EXCEPT:
    A. Carditis
    B. Fever

C. Chorea

D. Subcutaneous nodules

39. 62 year old, Mae F. complains of, "How can you help me? Hmmm, well, I have swallowing trouble, my young doctor, that's been bothering me a bit lately". She admits to slight weight loss, occasional heartburn and chest pain. Differential diagnosis would include:

    A. Esophageal cancer

    B. Gastroesophageal reflux

    C. Both

    D. Neither

40. Barium swallow reveals a large esophageal mass. Endoscopy reveals a large indurated ulcer in the lower third of the esophagus. Biopsies are obtained and reveal cancer. Which statement is true.

    A. The cancer is most probably a squamous cell and the prognosis is good to excellent with appropriate treatment.

    B. The cancer is most probably an adenocarcinoma and the prognosis is good to excellent with appropriate treatment.

    C. The cancer is most probably an adenocarcinoma and the prognosis is poor even with aggressive therapy.

    D. The cancer is most probably a squamous cell and the prognosis is poor even with aggressive therapy.

41. Complications of peptic ulcer disease include:

    A. Hemorrhage

    B. Perforation

    C. Obstruction

    D. Two of the above

    E. All of the above

42. All of the following are true statements concerning cancer of the stomach EXCEPT:

    A. Most lesions occur on the greater curvature

    B. Most lesions are adenocarcinomas

    C. There are few physical findings in early disease

    D. Gastric carcinoma is relatively radio-resistant

43. A 22 year old model returns from a "shoot" in Mexico. She complains of fever, chills, loose watery stools with both mucous and blood identified. She further complains of nausea, bloating and abdominal pain. Appropriate tests would include all of the following EXCEPT:

    A. CT of the abdomen

    B. Stool for blood, ova and parasites

    C. Fecal leukocytes

    D. Stool culture and sensitivity

    E. CBC

44. Giardia and pathogenic *E coli* are isolated. Appropriate therapy:

    A. Supportive therapy only

    B. Supportive therapy + metronidazole + ciprofloxacin

    C. Supportive therapy and oral vancomycin

    D. None of the above

45. An inflammatory bowel disease characterized by superficial inflammation of the colonic mucosa.

    A. Crohn's disease

    B. Irritable bowel syndrome

    C. Ulcerative colitis

    D. Diverticular disease

46. Complications of Crohn's disease include:

    A. Fistulas

    B. Intestinal obstruction

    C. Strictures

    D. Increased risk of colon cancer

    E. All of the above

47. A 48 year old man presents with LLQ pain and tenderness. He reports a change in bowel habit, and nausea over the last 24 hours. "Think it could be my appendix, doc?", he whispers.

Physical examination reveals fever to 100.5° F. recorded orally, LLQ pain with no guarding or rebound. There are decreased bowel sounds. CBC reveals a WBC count of 11,300 cell/mm³. The most likely diagnosis:
- A. Appendicitis
- B. Diverticulitis
- C. Irritable bowel syndrome
- D. None of the above

48. A 60 year old woman complains, "I just don't feel right after a movement, like I'm not quite done and I have to strain a bit." She also complains of vague abdominal and back pain. Guaiac is positive for occult blood and CBC reveals anemia. Barium enema reveals a mass in the descending colon. All of the following statements about colon cancer are true EXCEPT:
- A. 98% of adenocarcinomas of the colon are above the anal verge.
- B. Right-sided colon lesions are more common than left-sided lesions.
- C. About one-third of patients with colon cancer will present with metastases.
- D. The prognosis is poor.

49. 43 year old Fannie presents complaining, "Lord have mercy, I been sick with the nausea, the vomitin', the gas, and oh, how I bloat, with them fried foods, why I can't even have my ice cream no more and by the way, did I tell you... my right side hurts like, oh excuse me, you see, this belching I have...". The most probable diagnosis:
- A. Colon cancer
- B. Ulcerative colitis
- C. Peptic ulcer disease
- D. Irritable bowel syndrome
- E. None of the above

50. Which of the following statement(s) are true concerning hepatitis?

- A. Hepatitis A has no chronic form or carrier state
- B. Hepatitis B has a chronic form and a carrier state
- C. Hepatitis C is a major cause of post-transfusion hepatitis
- D. Two of the above
- E. All of the above

51. All of the following are predisposing factors to the development of hepatic carcinoma EXCEPT:
- A. Hepatitis A
- B. Hepatitis B
- C. Hepatitis C
- D. Cirrhosis

52. Which of the following statement(s) about acute pancreatitis are true?
- A. Approximately 80% of the cases are secondary to gallstones or ETOH abuse.
- B. There are elevations of the serum amylase and lipase
- C. Complications include pseudocysts, intra-abdominal infection and rarely hemorrhage.
- D. Two of the above
- E. All of the above

53. A 34 year old man presents with laboratory findings of proteinuria greater than 3.5 grams/day, hypo-albuminemia, edema, hyperlipidemia and lipiduria. The diagnosis:
- A. Acute nephritic syndrome
- B. Chronic nephritis
- C. Nephrotic syndrome
- D. Acute renal failure

54. Underlying cause(s) of chronic renal failure
- A. Diabetes mellitus
- B. Hypertension
- C. Glomerulonephritis
- D. Two of the above
- E. All of the above

55. Floyd T, a 46 year old male complains, "Feels like I got kicked in the back but can't tell what's worse, my back or this damn headache." Physical examination reveals a temperature of 101.5° F. recorded orally, CVA tenderness primarily left-sided, and lower back pain. Appropriate tests include all of the following EXCEPT:
    A. Urinalysis
    B. Urine culture and sensitivity
    C. CBC
    D. CT of the kidneys
    E. Blood cultures in severe disease

56. Statistically, the organism isolated from his urine:
    A. Enterococcus
    B. *Staphylococcus aureus*
    C. *E coli*
    D. *Proteus* sp.

57. Appropriate antibiotic therapy would include the use of:
    A. Trimethoprim-sulfamethoxazole
    B. Ciprofloxacin
    C. Amoxicillin or ampicillin
    D. Two of the above
    E. All of the above

58. The most common type of kidney stone:
    A. Struvite stones
    B. Calcium stones
    C. Uric acid stones
    D. Cystine stones

59. A 17 year old male presents with a three day history of dysuria associated with greenish-yellow urethral discharge. Gram stain reveals gram-negative intracellular diplococci within leukocytes. Culture is pending. The most likely diagnosis:
    A. *Neisseria gonorrhoeae*
    B. *Chlamydia trachomatis*
    C. *Treponema pallidum*
    D. *E coli*

60. This patient is allergic to penicillin. You would:
    A. Premedicate him with an antihistamine and try a small dose of penicillin to see if the patient reacts to it.
    B. Use ciprofloxacin 500 mg PO stat followed by seven days of doxycycline
    C. Trimethoprim-sulfamethoxazole
    D. Two of the above
    E. All of the above

61. A 23 year old woman is in tears as she complains of pain and labial swelling over the last 48 hours. Examination reveals grouped vesicles on an erythematous base. Painful ulcerations are also noted. The most probable diagnosis:
    A. Syphilis
    B. Condyloma lata
    C. *Herpes simplex* type 2
    D. *Trichomonal vaginitis*

62. Appropriate treatment of this illness:
    A. High dose penicillin therapy
    B. Podophyllin
    C. Acyclovir
    D. Metronidazole

63. You have initiated therapy on a 25 year old man diagnosed with secondary syphilis. Six hours after his injection with benzathine penicillin he develops fever, adenopathy, skin rash and arthralgias. You should:
    A. Discontinue all therapy immediately
    B. Discontinue the penicillin and begin doxycycline
    C. Continue therapy and monitor the patient
    D. None of the above

64. A 36 year old female presents complaining of postcoital spotting. Her pap smear is interpreted "class IV". You should:
    A. Follow the patient at yearly intervals
    B. Treat the patient for inflammatory changes on the cervix and repeat the pap smear in 3 months.

C. Inform the patient that she has an abnormal pap smear, that there may be malignant cells present, that more invasive testing is required and take immediate action.

D. Inform the patient that she has invasive carcinoma of the cervix and take immediate action

65. Histologic typing reveals most cervical cancers are:
    A. Adenocarcinomas
    B. Squamous cell carcinomas
    C. Adenosquamous carcinomas
    D. None of the above

66. "We've been trying so hard to have a baby", 27 year old Tammy T. cries softly as you speak to her. "Five years is a long, long time, and now this", she sobs. History reveals that she was told three weeks ago that she was pregnant at an AM-PM clinic. In the last 48 hours she's developed lower abdominal pain and has started vaginal spotting. You examine her and she is very tender over the area of the right tube and ovary and there may be some swelling. You repeat the urine β-hCG and it is positive. You should:

    A. Reassure the patient and send her home for strict bed rest.
    B. Treat her stat for probable PID
    C. Obtain a pelvic ultrasound, immediately
    D. Get a CT of the pelvis to work-up the probable ovarian mass

67. A 34 year old female presents stating, "I think I felt a lump in my right breast". You examine her and feel a 1 cm mass. There is no axillary adenopathy. You should:

    A. Reassure her that she has fibrocystic disease and recheck her in a year.
    B. Reassure her that the she has fibrocystic disease and recheck her in 6 months.
    C. Reassure her that the she has fibrocystic disease and recheck her in one month.
    D. Obtain a mammogram
    E. None of the above.

68. A mammogram:
    A. Can identify breast cancer 100% of the time
    B. Can identify and differentiate solid and cystic lesions
    C. Both statements are true
    D. Both statements are false

69. The active stage of labor is part of the:
    A. First stage of labor
    B. Second stage of labor
    C. Third stage of labor
    D. All of the above

70. With high-risk patients in the second stage of labor, fetal monitoring should be:
    A. Every thirty minutes
    B. After each contraction
    C. Continuous
    D. None of the above

71. A baby is born with an Apgar score of six at one minute and four at five minutes. Which statement is correct:
    A. The baby is off to a fine start and will do well without special care
    B. The baby is in distress and probably requires intensive care
    C. The baby needs immediate transfusion and treatment for severe Rh disease
    D. None of the above

72. A disease characterized by a symmetrical inflammatory polyarthritis:
    A. Osteoarthritis
    B. Gouty arthritis
    C. Rheumatoid arthritis
    D. Systemic lupus erythematosus

73. Examination of the synovial fluid from a swollen knee joint reveals normal fluid color, viscosity, negative mucin clot test, WBCs of 200 cells/ mm³ and wear and mineral particles.

Based on this information, the most likely diagnosis:
    A. Gouty arthritis
    B. Rheumatoid arthritis
    C. Systemic lupus erythematosus
    D. Osteoarthritis

74.   47 year old Besty R. is "nervous" complaining of "this rash on my face that, oh, I almost forgot, I can't even go in the sun any more and look, look here at my mouth, these ulcers, and I just can't get my work done like I've done for years and I feel terrible, just terrible with my fingers aching, and the fever at night and Louis, he's my husband, tells me I'm losing weight and you know here lately, I just eat like a bird..." Based on the information above, probable laboratory results would include:
    A. Positive ANA
    B. Positive Ph^1 chromosome
    C. Positive Bence-Jones protein
    D. None of the above

75.   "Think I got me a bladder problem, here doc", drawls Jimmy T. a 35 year old farmer. "I just keep a goin' and goin' like I got nothin' better to do out in there in the fields. And thirsty, powerful thirsty out there in the sun, parched-like and hungry, like I'm an 18 year old buck again but losin' my weight. Based on the information above, probable laboratory results would include:
    A. Abnormal CT of the chest
    B. Positive rheumatoid factor
    C. Elevated PSA
    D. None of the above

76.   The most probable diagnosis:
    A. Lung cancer
    B. Rheumatoid arthritis
    C. Prostatic cancer causing post-renal obstruction
    D. None of the above

77.   Andy B., a 30 year old dental student presents with nervousness, fatigue, weakness, weight loss, palpitations, tremor, frequency of bowel movements, emotional lability and proptosis. Based on the

information above, probable laboratory results would include:
    A. No laboratory abnormality
    B. Elevated T_4, elevated FTI, and TSH suppression
    C. Abnormal echocardiogram of the heart
    D. None of the above

78.   The most probable diagnosis:
    A. Agitated depression
    B. Hyperthyroidism
    C. Restricted cardiomyopathy
    D. None of the above

79.   Treatment would consist of:
    A. Out-patient psychotherapy and placement on antidepressants.
    B. Radioactive iodine followed by thyroid replacement
    C. Anticoagulation, antiarrhythmics and possible heart transplantation.
    D. None of the above

80.   "Cold nodules" of the thyroid gland are:
    A. Functional
    B. Nonfunctional
    C. Usually malignant
    D. Usually benign
    E. A and C
    F. B and D

81.   A history of back pain, decreasing height, dowager's hump and fractures with no significant trauma in a 68 year old woman is most consistent with:
    A. Multiple myeloma
    B. Osteoarthritis
    C. Osteoporosis
    D. Hypothyroidism

82.   "I don't like to complain sir, but my big toe feels like it is on fire", sighed the 39 year old, tight-lipped accountant. Based on the information above, probable laboratory results would include:
    A. Elevated uric acid
    B. Elevated calcium

C. Abnormal "M" proteins

D. None of the above

83. The most likely diagnosis:

    A. Gout

    B. Hyperparathyroidism

    C. Multiple myeloma

    D. None of the above

84. A cholesterol of 300 mg/dL is classified as:

    A. Normal

    B. Mild hypercholesterolemia

    C. Moderate hypercholesterolemia

    D. Severe hypercholesterolemia

85. Sophie Y., a 34 year old woman who just had a major argument with her husband, presents with scotomas associated with visual field loss, and mood changes followed by a severe unilateral headache. The most probable diagnosis:

    A. Common migraine headache

    B. Cluster headache

    C. Tension headache

    D. None of the above

86. A three year old boy, Ricky Z., presents two weeks after a sinus infection which really "just took care of itself". He is diaphoretic, has a rectal temperature of 104.5° F., and is chilling. He complains of headache and photophobia. His mother stated he vomited on the way to your office. On physical examination he is lethargic and has meningismus. While you are examining him he has a seizure. The most probable diagnosis:

    A. Idiopathic seizure disorder

    B. CNS tumor

    C. Meningitis

    D. Severe sinus infection

87. The seizure ends abruptly and you advise the mother to:

    A. Take him to the hospital for an EEG

    B. Take him to the hospital for a CT scan

    C. Take him to the hospital for admission and IV antibiotics

    D. Take him home and treat him as an outpatient with oral antibiotics

88. The majority of adult CNS tumors are located:

    A. Supratentorial

    B. Posterior fossa

    C. Brain stem

    D. None of the above

89. All of the following are true EXCEPT:

    A. A glioblastoma multiforme is an astrocytoma grade 3 or 4

    B. An acoustic neuroma is a curable tumor

    C. The medulloblastoma is a relatively common adult and a relatively uncommon childhood tumor

    D. None of the above

90. The classification of stroke by percentage of cases:

    A. Ischemic stroke = hemorrhagic stroke

    B. Ischemic stroke > hemorrhagic stroke

    C. Ischemic stroke < hemorrhagic stroke

    D. None of the above

91. A hypochromic, microcytic anemia:

    A. Iron deficiency anemia

    B. Megaloblastic anemia

    C. Both

    D. Neither

92. A patient is diagnosed with chronic myelogenous leukemia. You would expect:

    A. The presence of Auer rods

    B. The presence of the Ph^1 chromosome

    C. The malignant proliferation of abnormal B-cell lymphocytes

    D. Malignant proliferation of an early hematopoietic precursor yielding immature lymphoid cells referred to as blasts.

93. A 60 year old man complains, "My bones ache like never before, you see, doc, my arthritis is just getting worse, I guess". He also complains of fatigue, weight loss and "black and blue marks all over my body".

He hands you X-rays his chiropractor sent for you to evaluate. They reveal multiple lytic bone lesions. You would expect:

    A. The presence of Auer rods

    B. The presence of increased mature lymphocytes in the marrow

    C. Serum and/or urine monoclonal (M) protein and marrow plasma cells greater than 10%

    D. The presence of Reed-Sternberg cells in a lymph node biopsy

94.   The Reed-Sternberg cell:

    A. Can be identified in chronic myelo-genous leukemia

    B. Can be identified in acute myelogenous leukemia

    C. Is pathognomonic for multiple myeloma

    D. None of the above

95.   Treatment of Hodgkin's disease may include:

    A. Surgery for biopsy and staging laparotomy

    B. Radiation therapy

    C. Chemotherapy

    D. All of the above

    E. None of the above

96.   "I just don't know, doc, I think I got the flu when I was hunting three days ago.", says 32 year old Ralph K. "Low-grade fever and chills and my muscles ache like hell. And hey, now look at this rash on my hands and feet that came out this morning." Physical examination reveals a temperature of 100 °F recorded orally, a petechial rash which now involves the arms and legs. There is a small sore on the lower leg and when you question Ralph he says, "Burned the head of a tick there yesterday. The CBC is normal. You would:

    A. Treat for flu and contact dermatitis

    B. Treat for staphylococcal cellulitis

    C. Treat for secondary syphilis

    D. None of the above

97.   Koplik's spots:

    A. Rubella

    B. Varicella

    C. Mumps

    D. None of the above

98.   The etiology of mononucleosis:

    A. A bacteria

    B. A fungus

    C. A parasite

    D. None of the above

99.   The presence of increased levels of cortisol:

    A. Acromegaly

    B. Gigantism

    C. Addison's disease

    D. None of the above

100.   AIDS:

    A. Predisposes patients to opportunistic infections.

    B. Can be spread by casual contact.

    C. Both statements are true

    D. Both statements are false

ANSWERS TO SELF-ASSESSMENT EXAMINATION

1. C	26. D	51. A	76. D
2. C	27. D	52. E	77. B
3. C	28. C	53. C	78. B
4. B	29. C	54. E	79. B
5. A	30. A	55. D	80. F
6. D	31. E	56. C	81. C
7. C	32. A	57. D	82. A
8. A	33. C	58. B	83. A
9. B	34. A	59. A	84. D
10. D	35. E	60. B	85. A
11. D	36. B	61. C	86. C
12. A	37. D	62. C	87. C
13. B	38. B	63. C	88. A
14. A	39. C	64. C	89. C
15. E	40. D	65. B	90. B
16. B	41. E	66. C	91. A
17. D	42. A	67. D	92. B
18. C	43. A	68. D	93. C
19. E	44. B	69. A	94. D
20. D	45. C	70. C	95. D
21. E	46. E	71. B	96. D
22. A	47. B	72. C	97. D
23. A	48. B	73. D	98. D
24. D	49. E	74. A	99. D
25. A	50. E	75. D	100. A